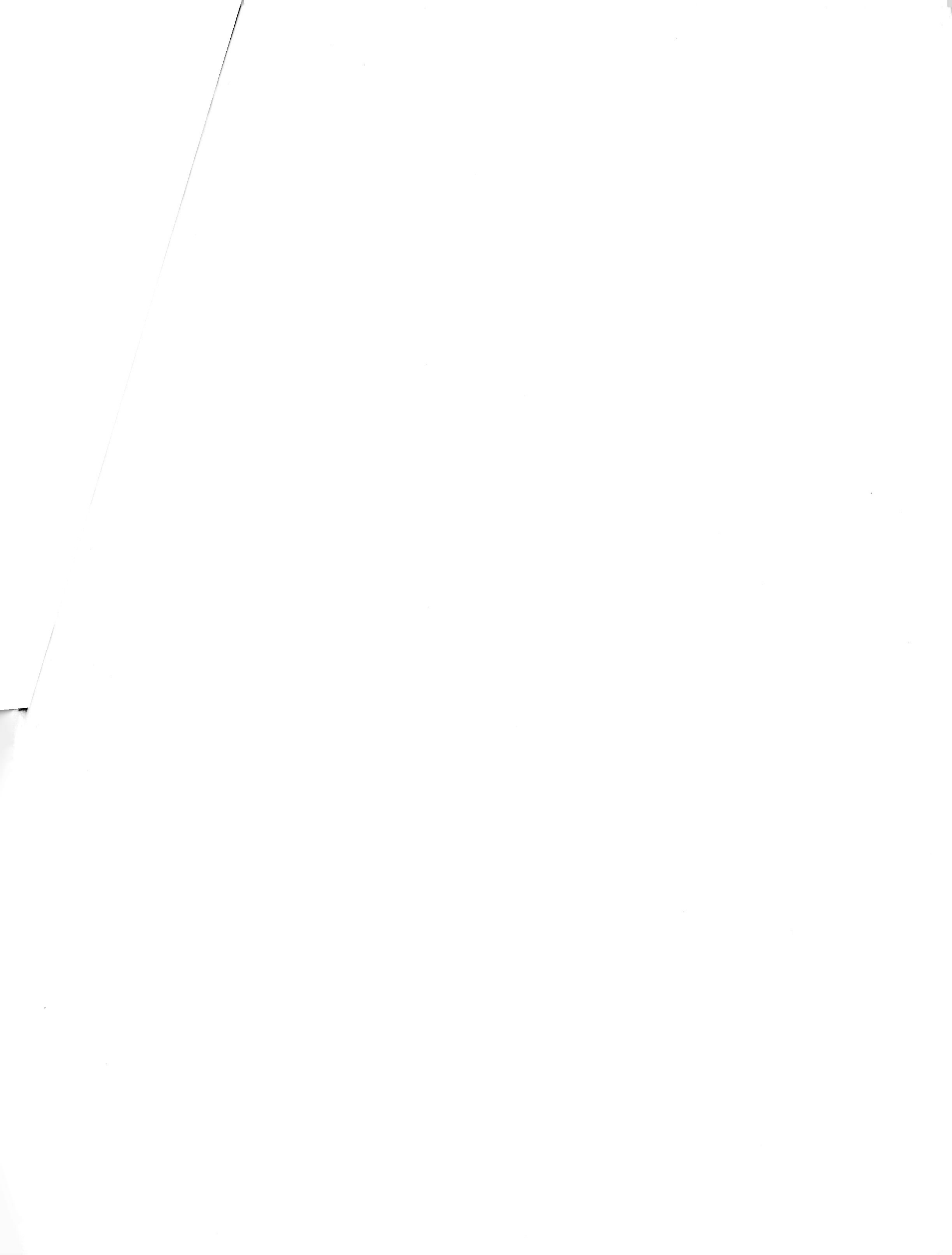

A Color Atlas of Morphologic Hematology

A Color Atlas of Morphologic Hematology

WITH A GUIDE TO CLINICAL INTERPRETATION

BY

GENEVA A. DALAND, B.S.

CHIEF LABORATORY ASSISTANT IN HEMATOLOGY, THORNDIKE MEMORIAL LABORATORY
RESEARCH LABORATORY TECHNICIAN, BOSTON CITY HOSPITAL

EDITED BY

THOMAS HALE HAM, M.D.

PROFESSOR OF MEDICINE AND CHAIRMAN OF THE COMMITTEE ON MEDICAL EDUCATION
WESTERN RESERVE UNIVERSITY, SCHOOL OF MEDICINE, CLEVELAND, OHIO

ILLUSTRATIONS BY

ETTA PIOTTI

REVISED EDITION

HARVARD UNIVERSITY PRESS—CAMBRIDGE, MASSACHUSETTS

1965

PRINTED IN THE UNITED STATES OF AMERICA

Second Printing

DISTRIBUTED IN GREAT BRITAIN BY
OXFORD UNIVERSITY PRESS, LONDON

Plate II is reproduced from J. L. Bremer and Harold L. Weatherford, Textbook of histology *(ed. 6), copyright 1936, 1944 by The Blakiston Company, by permission of the publisher.*

Plate I and Plates III through IX are reproduced from Nelson's Loose-Leaf Medicine, *vol. 4, copyright 1940 by Thomas Nelson & Sons, by permission of the publisher.*

PREFACE

The purpose of this *Atlas* is to furnish a guide for reference in the study of films of peripheral blood stained with Wright's stain. The description of the blood, in a variety of clinical conditions, is considered from a diagnostic point of view. The maturation of the blood cells is described and shown in the diagrams and plates so that immature or abnormal forms may be recognized in the peripheral blood or bone marrow. It is emphasized that these diagrams are oversimplified for use as working hypotheses by those who are concerned with diagnosis and treatment. No attempt is made to discuss in detail the many theories regarding the origin of the cells or to show, in the diagrams, other possible concepts. The terminology used or the theories of cell origin are not as important as the recognition of the significance of the findings from a diagnostic, prognostic, and therapeutic point of view. The morphology of cells of the bone marrow is not discussed separately, since cells of the bone marrow may appear in the peripheral blood in certain physiologic or pathologic conditions. The details of quantitative methods, special tests, as well as physiologic and pathologic aspects of the diseases involving red cells, white cells, and platelets are given in *A syllabus of laboratory examinations in clinical diagnosis* [116], which is a companion book of this *Atlas*.

The author is indebted to the late Dr. George R. Minot whose guidance and enthusiasm were enjoyed for many years. The constant encouragement, support, and guidance of Dr. William B. Castle and Dr. Thomas Hale Ham have made progress in this field possible. The author wishes to acknowledge also the assistance and counsel given by Dr. Frederic Parker, Jr., and Dr. Henry Jackson, Jr., not only in the preparation of this volume, but in the study of the morphology of the blood and the pathology of many unusual cases over many years.

The value of this book is largely due to the excellent drawings by Etta Piotti, whose untimely death occurred since her work for this volume was completed.

G. A. D.

CONTENTS

PLATES

following page 72

FIGURES

TABLES

A Color Atlas of Morphologic Hematology

1. VALUE AND LIMITATIONS OF THE BLOOD FILM IN DIAGNOSIS

1. *DETECTION OF ABNORMALITIES OF FORMED ELEMENTS BY BRIEF SCREENING EXAMINATION.* A brief but critical screening examination of the blood film stained with Wright's stain is an essential part of the complete examination of each patient. Abnormalities of the red cells, the white cells, and the platelets can be detected rapidly by inspection. If abnormalities are apparent, other examinations are indicated, such as red-cell count, determination of the red-cell indices of Wintrobe, reticulocyte count, white-cell count, platelet count, bone-marrow aspirations, and other special tests discussed in the *Syllabus* [116]. The variation of the red cells from normal is observed in respect to their size, shape, and hemoglobin content, and the presence of abnormal forms, as discussed in Sec. 5 and shown in Plate I, is noted. It is usually possible to estimate whether the white-cell count is normal, increased, or decreased. An important observation is the deviation from the normal proportion of white cells, as shown by neutrophilia, lymphocytosis, monocytosis, eosinophilia, neutropenia, or lymphopenia. The finding of immature cells or of cells not normally seen in the peripheral blood is of great importance. Slight variations from the normal in the number of platelets observed in a blood film are of little clinical significance. However, the absence of platelets or a definite decrease in their number may indicate a primary or secondary thrombocytopenia. The presence of large or abnormal platelets may indicate a fundamental disturbance of the bone marrow.

2. *EVALUATION OF THE ACTIVITY OF THE BONE MARROW FROM EXAMINATION OF THE PERIPHERAL BLOOD.* The degree of activity of the bone marrow in the production of formed elements may be evident in the film of peripheral blood. For example, all the formed elements may be decreased in the peripheral blood; this condition is described by the term pancytopenia. The presence of moderate numbers of polychromatophilic macrocytes in a blood film showing normochromic or hypochromic red cells suggests the recent occurrence of blood loss and a physiologic response of the bone marrow. The occurrence of polychromatophilic cells in large numbers in chronic anemia, with icterus, with or without spheroidal red cells, strongly suggests a hemolytic anemia. Examination of the blood film is of value in determining the response, or lack of response, of pernicious anemia and the related macrocytic anemias to vitamin B_{12} (liver extract), or of hypochromic iron-deficient anemia to the administration of iron. The presence of polychromatophilic cells or, better, the actual number of reticulocytes, indicates the degree of erythropoietic activity of the bone marrow.

3. *CONFIRMATION OF A DIAGNOSIS OR SUPPLEMENTING OTHER DATA.* There are many instances in clinical medicine in which data from the blood film aid in confirming a diagnosis or supplement other data available to the physician. Thus, the identification of the abnormal cells characteristic of infectious mononucleosis aids materially in distinguishing it from the fatal disease, leukemia. Also, the blood film is essential for the establishment of a clinical diagnosis of malaria, Oroya fever, and certain other parasitic diseases. Most pyogenic infections are associated with leukocytosis and neutrophilia, whereas leukopenia or neutropenia may occur in such infections as typhoid fever, brucellosis, and virus infections. The presence of eosinophilia may suggest a diagnosis of trichinosis.

2. PREPARATION OF BLOOD FILMS

A thin, well-stained film of blood is essential for the critical evaluation of the blood cells. The blood film should be thin enough that the red cells do not overlap and that the white cells are spread out for observation of details of the nuclear structure, color of the cytoplasm, type of granules, and relative size of the cell.

For successful preparation of films of blood, the slides or coverglasses must be washed free from acid and alkali, which alter the staining reaction, and free from grease, which interferes with uniform spreading of the blood film. For the most accurate results, the differential count of white cells should be made on a stained film prepared on a coverglass (No. 0 or No. 1, $\frac{7}{8}$ inch square). In such films, the blood spreads by capillary action and the dispersion of the leukocytes is that of a chance distribution [13, 116]. In slide preparations the distribution of leukocytes is not uniform, since the large red and white cells accumulate in increased numbers along the edge and at the end of the blood film. Slide preparations are preferred for the work in parasitology, where a thick drop and a thin film may be prepared on the same slide.

1. *SOURCE OF THE SPECIMEN.* When a sample of venous blood is taken for blood counts a small drop of blood from the tip of the needle is placed on a coverglass and covered with another coverglass held in such a position as to form with the first an eight-pointed star. As soon as the drop of blood has spread over the surface, the coverglasses are separated by sliding the upper one off of the lower one, holding them in the same plane in which they are lying. Coverglasses should never be separated by lifting. Preparations are air dried and placed vertically in a box with slits or partitions.

For some purposes capillary blood is sufficient or preferred. A sterile instrument for puncturing the lobe of the ear or the tip of the finger should always be used, and should always be resterilized before being used again. The Fenwal lancets, hemolets, or a No. 11 Bard-Parker blade have been found to be satisfactory. Obtaining the blood sample from the ear is preferred to obtaining it from the finger because it causes less discomfort to the patient and is less likely to lead to infection. It has been found, however, that the white-cell count in blood from the ear is normally slightly greater than in that from the finger [59, 177] and that large white cells may be present in greater numbers. This may be a distinct advantage in the study of the blood in bacterial endocarditis, infectious mononucleosis, leukopenia, and leukemia. Blood samples from the finger give results comparable to those in the venous sample. The red-cell counts and hemoglobin are essentially the same in the samples from the ear as in those from the finger and the vein. In children blood is usually collected from the finger if it is not possible or necessary to obtain a venous sample. In infants, the puncture is usually made in the heel.

In an emergency, blood films may be made from samples of venous blood containing anticoagulants, but they are not satisfactory for the morphologic study of white cells, since white cells change in their staining characteristics, develop vacuoles, phagocytose crystals of oxalate, and degenerate gradually on standing. As a result, the nucleus of the lymphocyte may appear to be dividing, the nucleus of the monocyte often appears as a clover leaf, and the lobes of the neutrophil are often separated into distinct parts.

2. *PRINCIPLES AND METHODS OF STAINING THE BLOOD FILM.*

WRIGHT'S STAIN. Wright's stain, a common modification of the Romanowsky stain, is a combination of methylene blue, methylene azure, and eosin. As stated by Conn [49], " these compound dyes act on the protoplasm somewhat as follows: certain parts of the cell have an affinity for the neutral stain and take it up as such; others, having an affinity for the basic dye, break up the neutral stain so as to obtain the basic portion of it, or, if dissociation has taken place, take up the basic ion directly; while other parts of the cell with an affinity for acid dyes similarly combine with the acid portion of the stain." The nucleus of the cells, or especially the chromatin within the nuclei, is assumed to be acid in character (owing largely to the constituent nucleic acid), has an affinity for a basic dye (methylene blue), and is termed basophilic. Neutral material is stained violet in color and is termed neutrophilic. Basic material is stained by an acid dye (eosin) and is termed eosinophilic. Azurophilic, as the name implies, indicates an affinity for methylene azure, which is red-purple.

Wright's stain, certified by the Commission on Staining [49], may be purchased in solution or in powdered form. The solution is prepared by dissolving 0.1 gm of powder in 60 ml of absolute methyl alcohol (acetone-free and chemically pure). The stain should be filtered when made and whenever samples are taken from the stock solution. Care should be taken to keep the reagent bottles stoppered, and to avoid contamination with water or acid.

The buffer solution for use in diluting the Wright's stain should have a pH of 6.4 to 6.8. A phosphate buffer solution with pH 6.7 may be prepared by mixing 43.5 ml of M/15 anhydrous secondary sodium phosphate (Na_2HPO_4, 9.47 gm/lit) and 56.5 ml of M/15 primary potassium phosphate (KH_2PO_4, 9.08 gm/lit).

The coverglasses, preferably with fresh but dry blood films, are placed in a horizontal position on a flat support or a rubber stopper and covered with Wright's stain. After remaining for 3 min. the stain is diluted with an approximately equal volume of buffer or tap water and allowed to stain for another 3 min. The pH of the diluting fluid should be 6.4 to 6.8; distilled water is often too acid. The stain is then floated off by holding the coverglass in a horizontal plane under the running tap water for a short time. The preparation is then dried thoroughly by careful blotting with filter paper. When dry, any extra stain on the back of the coverglass is removed with gauze moistened in alcohol. The dry coverglass preparations are mounted, with the blood film face down, on a clean glass slide on which has been placed a drop of isobutyl methacrylate dissolved in xylol. The mounting fluid should be in the same pH range (6.4 to 6.8) as the stain. When an acid mounting fluid is used the staining of the cells on the films deteriorates with time. Enough mounting fluid should be used to spread completely over the surface and air bubbles should be avoided. For satisfactory staining and preservation of blood films contamination with acid or acid fumes should be avoided throughout the procedure. Evaporation of the alcohol of the stain during the procedure causes undesirable precipitate and often produces a muddy background.

Brilliant Cresyl Blue for Reticulocytes. Brilliant cresyl blue is used as a vital stain to precipitate the basophilic substance of the red cells, which appears polychromatophilic when stained only with Wright's stain. The cells containing this precipitated basophilic substance are called reticulocytes. Counts may be performed on fresh preparations or permanent preparations counterstained with Wright's stain. Whatever method is chosen for a particular study should be used throughout the investigation to assure comparable results. Prolonged contact of the dye with the cells will give slightly higher values for reticulocytes than a brief exposure. The advantage of the permanent preparation can be readily appreciated, since the counts do not have to be made immediately and the slides may be filed for reference. In reticulocyte preparations the basophilic substance of the white cells is also precipitated in the cytoplasm, so that differentiation of the white cells is sometimes difficult. Such preparations should be used for a differential white-cell count only when plain, Wright's-stained films are not available.

For the permanent preparations an alcoholic solution of brilliant cresyl blue is used. It is made by dissolving 0.5 gm of brilliant cresyl blue in 100 ml of 95-percent ethyl alcohol. This is a saturated solution and should be filtered when made up and each time aliquots are taken from the stock solution for the preparation of cresyl blue coverglasses. Evaporation of the stock solution will cause precipitation of the stain.

Preparation of the cresyl blue coverglasses requires the use of coverglasses that have been carefully cleaned and dried. Coverglasses are usually left for several hours in cleaning solution (potassium dichromate and sulfuric acid) or in soap and water. They should then be rinsed thoroughly until the rinse water gives a neutral reaction to litmus. The coverglasses are then stored in alcohol until dried for use. The coverglasses are placed on a flat surface and just enough (1 or 2 drops) of the alcoholic solution of brilliant cresyl blue is added to cover the surface of each coverglass. These are covered with a glass beaker or cover to reduce the rate of evaporation of the alcohol. When dry, the stained surface appears gray. The coverglass is polished until a purple color is obtained by rubbing lightly, stain side down, on a smooth or glazed paper. These prepared coverslips are stored, stained surfaces together, until needed. A convenient rack may be made by cutting slits in the cover of a cardboard box in which the corners of the coverglasses may be placed.

The reticulocytes are stained by placing a drop of blood on the stained surface of one of these previously prepared coverglasses. A second coverglass, stained surface down, is placed crosswise on the drop of blood, making an eight-pointed star. When the blood has spread over the entire surface, by capillarity, not pressure, the two coverglasses should be separated by sliding them apart promptly and in the same plane in which they are lying. When the films are dry, they should be counterstained with Wright's stain.

3. *EXAMINATION OF THE QUALITY OF THE STAINED BLOOD FILM.* A general survey of the blood film should be made, using the high dry objective of the microscope, to judge the quality of the film. In most fields examined, the red cells and white cells should be clearly separated, should show no artifacts such as vacuoles in the red cells, and should not show significant amounts of precipitate. The staining should be uniform throughout. The stain should be alkaline enough to stain clearly the platelets, polychromatophilic cells, granules in the neutrophilic series, stippled cells, and the nuclei of the cells, and acid enough to bring out the contrast between the nuclei and the cytoplasm of neutrophils.

The optimum pH is about 6.4 to 6.8 for the buffer solution used in diluting the Wright's stain on the film. Excessive red staining or red areas are due to an acid reaction. This might be caused by acid fumes while staining, coverglasses that were not thoroughly rinsed, or areas that were still moist when the coverglass was mounted. Excessive blue staining may be due to alkali, to excessive thickness of the film, or to evaporation of the alcoholic stain and drying of the film. In thick films, when the red cells are piled up, the cytoplasm of the white cells will be condensed about the nucleus so that structure cannot be observed and the granules are not distinct enough to be identified.

The distribution of the cells should be uniform, without a concentration of cells at one end or around the periphery. This condition is difficult to obtain in the slide preparation. Precipitate on the film interferes with the recognition of platelets and reticulocytes and may be avoided by floating off the precipitate formed in staining, by thorough washing of the films, and by filtering the stain frequently. The presence of small bubblelike deformities of the surface of the red cells is an artifact indicating that the film was mounted before being thoroughly dried. The mounting medium, preferably methacrylate, should spread beneath the entire film, since air pockets interfere with clear definition of the cells. If the stained blood film is unsatisfactory, it is a waste of time to examine it in detail, since the results are unreliable and may be seriously misleading. Another blood film should be prepared.

3. PREPARATION OF THE COLOR PLATES

1. *USE OF WRIGHT'S STAIN IN THIS* ATLAS. The films of peripheral blood reproduced in this *Color atlas* were stained with Wright's stain. Although this is a limited method of study, it is of practical value, since Wright's stain is widely used in clinical medicine. Accordingly, the color values and descriptions in this book are limited to those obtained by using Wright's stain and brilliant cresyl blue. The structure of the cells as described results in part from fixation by methyl alcohol contained in Wright's stain. The color of the stained cells is an expression of the affinity of the cellular elements for the acid, basic, or neutral portions of this stain. Other methods of staining, such as supravital staining, the peroxidase stain, and histochemical methods, are of value in special instances [116]).

2. *PREPARATION AND USE OF THE COLOR PLATES.* The cells in the color plates (Plates I to XVI) were drawn using a camera lucida and painted in water color as they were observed through the microscope with a magnification of 1200. Each plate represents a composite of two or three oil-immersion fields from blood films of patients with proved diagnoses. In these plates will be found the cells that occur in peripheral blood in the normal subject, as well as most of the progenitors of blood cells. The immature

forms that normally are found in bone marrow or other tissues may occur in the peripheral blood in abnormal states. Thus, the identification of cells in these plates of peripheral blood will aid in performing differential cell counts of aspirations of bone marrow. The plates are limited in number and represent conditions in which the film of blood is of definite diagnostic value. Emphasis is placed on the interpretation of the cells found in these films and on the differential diagnosis of the conditions in which related abnormalities may be found.

4. GENERAL CHARACTERISTICS OF FORMED ELEMENTS OF BLOOD STAINED WITH WRIGHT'S STAIN

1. *CHARACTERISTICS OF THE CELL.* The formed elements of the blood include the nucleated red cells and white cells, the nonnucleated mature red cells, and the platelets. The cytoplasm, enclosed in cell membrane, may appear clear or may contain granules, rods, or foreign particles that have been phagocytosed. The nucleus of white cells and of nucleated red cells contains a network of chromatin material, and, in the primitive cells, one or more nucleoli may be present within the nucleus. With Wright's stain, the nucleolus appears as a circumscribed area, about 2 to 3 μ in diameter, that is less densely stained than the surrounding nucleus. In films stained with brilliant cresyl blue, the nucleolus appears as a light-blue area. Nucleoli should be distinguished from dark-staining clumps of chromatin and from vacuoles, which may appear as clear colorless areas of variable size and number in either the nucleus or the cytoplasm of the cell. Films that have been stored for years sometimes show degenerative changes or clear areas in the nuclear chromatin that are not nucleoli. In films of bone-marrow aspirations or in the peripheral blood in the leukemias, nuclear division or mitosis may be seen.

2. *IDENTIFICATION OF CELLS.* For study and identification of the cells in a film of blood it is essential to examine the preparation with oil-immersion magnification (1000 to 1200) and adequate illumination. It is necessary not only to see the cells but to " see the inside of the cells," to study the color of the granules and the details of the structure of the nucleus. The variation in types of blood cells is great. Cells may be identified as belonging to the red-cell series, the white-cell series, or the thrombocytic series. Further classification of the white cells may be made by grouping them into the granulocytic, lymphocytic, monocytic, plasmacytic, or histiocytic series. To understand the different cells in each series, the several stages of development of the cell must be appreciated (see Figs. 4, 5, 6, 7, 9). These stages may be seen in aspirations of bone marrow, and also in the peripheral blood in certain infections and in anemia and leukemia. The degree of immaturity of the blood cells seen in the peripheral blood is a rough index of the physiologic response of the bone marrow or other tissues, or may indicate abnormal growth, as in neoplastic diseases. The appearance of abortive types of cells is also a sign of abnormality that may have a serious prognosis. Such cells may be present in a terminal illness, in overwhelming sepsis, or after prolonged irradiation.

An accurate report of the blood findings on the part of the technologist is important. An understanding of these abnormal cells and their significance is equally important for the physician, in order that he may interpret the physiologic and pathologic significance of the laboratory data.

If a cell is difficult to classify, it should be compared with cells that can be recognized for the structure of the nucleus, the color and structure of the cytoplasm, and the type and color of the granules. If a cell cannot be recognized as belonging to any of the established series, it should be recorded as an abnormal cell and described in detail, with a drawing.

Cell development can be described in a systematic manner, since the morphologic changes are similar in some respects for each series of cells described here. Some generalizations will be helpful in studying the cells, although there are many exceptions to all the rules that can be established. Differentiation of the type and age of the cells must be determined by a consideration of many factors. Some of these factors are size, structure of the nucleus, color of nuclear chromatin, presence of nucleoli, character and color of the cytoplasm, relative proportion of nucleus and cytoplasm, granulation, and color of the granules. No one factor can be considered alone, although the structure of the nucleus is probably the most valuable single guide.

(*a*) Relative Size of Cells. In general, immature cells are larger than mature cells. The stem cell is definitely larger than the other blasts of any series (Figs. 1, 4, 5, 6, 7, and 9). Other examples may be seen by comparing the proerythroblast with the normoblast, the polychromatophilic cell with the mature red cell (Fig. 1), and the myelocyte with the mature granulocyte (Fig. 4). Abnormal eosinophils in infectious states are usually larger than the normal eosinophil. In infections the myelocytes and band forms are larger than the neutrophils, and the neutrophils may be larger than those in normal blood. The mature small lymphocyte is the smallest cell of the white-cell series. The plasmablast and the young plasma cell are larger than the mature plasma cell, although the mature cell may be large in the leukemic states.

(*b*) Relative Size of Nucleus and Cytoplasm. The nucleus in the immature cell takes up a larger proportion of the cell than it does in the mature cell. Examples of this are especially striking in the granulocytic series (Fig. 4). In the lymphocytic series (Fig. 5) this generalization holds except for the small lymphocyte, in which the nucleus occupies most of the cell.

(*c*) Nuclear Structure as a Distinguishing Characteristic. The characteristics of the nuclear structure are illustrated diagrammatically in Figs. 1, 4, 5, 6, 7, 8, 9 and in more exact detail in the color plates (I through XVI). These details are realized most effectively if the observer reproduces the cells on paper either with pencil or with colored crayons.

In general, the young cells have a uniformly granular structure of the chromatin of the nucleus, while the mature forms of each series are characterized by a heavy condensation of chromatin, as is seen in the small lymphocyte, plasma cell, neutrophil, and normoblast. However, the monocyte and histiocyte are definitely exceptions to this generalization. The color of the nuclei of the mature cells in general is blue-purple, and is more intense than the red-purple of the blast nuclei. Nucleoli are present in the youngest forms. It is of utmost importance to differentiate the blast from other cells by careful observation of the type of the nucleus. The series to which a blast cell belongs is determined in part by the size of the cell, the color of the cytoplasm, and the structure of the nucleus as compared with other blasts, and in part by the presence of other cells of the same series ("by the company they keep"). Blasts from more than one series may be present, as, for example, granulocytic and erythrocytic series. See also pp. 26, 35, 39, 40, Plates V, VII, VIII, XI.

(*d*) Color of the Cytoplasm as a Differential Criterion. The stem cell, the proerythroblast, and all the blasts of the white-cell series are characterized by the deep basophilia of the cytoplasm, although the shade and character of this deep blue varies somewhat in the different series. The proerythroblast has a gray-blue cytoplasm, somewhat similar to that of the monoblast. The cytoplasm of the myeloblast is usually rather a clear deep blue, but is more abundant than that of the lymphoblast.

The change from the deep basophilia of the proerythroblast to the hemoglobin-containing cytoplasm of the normoblast and the mature erythrocyte may be seen diagrammatically in Fig. 1 and in Plate I. In the intermediate stages both elements — the basophilic substance and the hemoglobin — are factors in producing the polychromatophilia of the cytoplasm, the relative amount of each substance determining the intensity of the color. As the cell matures, basophilic substance decreases and hemoglobin increases.

The disappearance of the basophilic substance as the cell matures is illustrated in the granulocytic series by comparison of the cytoplasm of myelocyte A with that of myelocyte C (Plate XI).

In the lymphocytic series the mature small lymphocyte and the large lymphocyte have the lightest-blue cytoplasm of any of the blood cells. However, the young lymphocyte has practically as blue a cytoplasm as the lymphoblast. Some small lymphocytes do have deep-blue cytoplasm, which

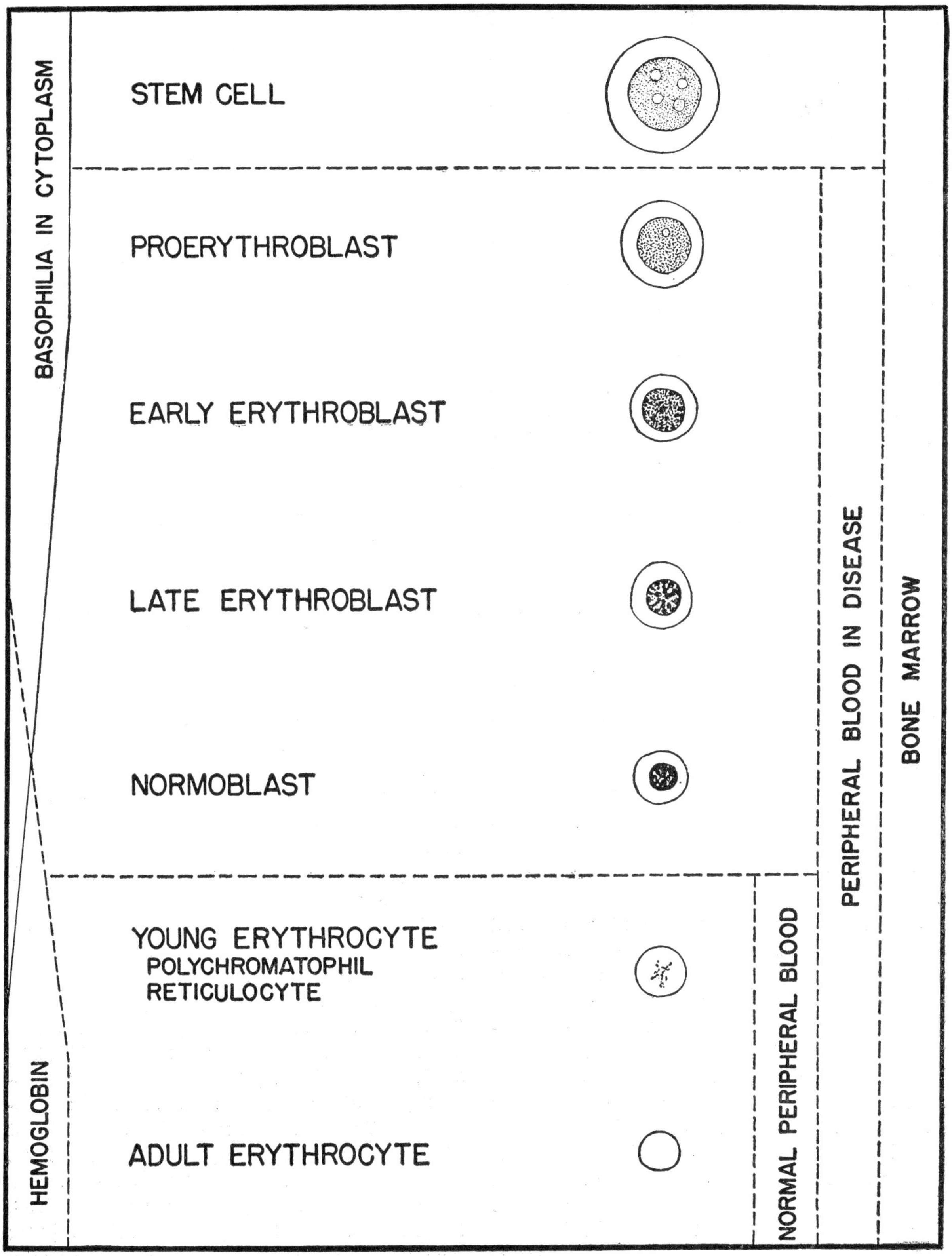

BASOPHILIA IN CYTOPLASM

STEM CELL

PROERYTHROBLAST

EARLY ERYTHROBLAST

LATE ERYTHROBLAST

NORMOBLAST

YOUNG ERYTHROCYTE
POLYCHROMATOPHIL
RETICULOCYTE

ADULT ERYTHROCYTE

HEMOGLOBIN

NORMAL PERIPHERAL BLOOD

PERIPHERAL BLOOD IN DISEASE

BONE MARROW

FIG. 1. Diagram of the maturation of the erythrocytic series.

may be due to a crowded area in the film with resulting condensation of the cytoplasm about the nucleus, or they may be young forms, according to the studies of Wiseman [308]. If the films are thick, it is difficult to tell the lymphocyte from the monocyte because the details of the cytoplasm cannot be seen. The mature plasma cell has a deep-blue cytoplasm which is usually less intense than the blast of the same series.

(*e*) Color Values. Use of the compound, polychromatic, Romanowsky stains, such as Wright's stain [49], affords the advantage of staining the acidophilic and basophilic elements at the same time. This actually means that there is a gradation of staining reaction from the deep blue (acid in reaction but " basophilic " in staining) of the cytoplasm of the blast to the red (basic in reaction but " acidophilic " in staining) of the mature red cell. This gradation in color value applies to the nucleus, to the cytoplasm, and to the granules and may be more clearly understood from the systematic color scheme shown in Fig. 2. In this chart the color relations of the cellular elements of the blood (nucleus, cytoplasm, and granules) are shown graphically in a color circle. Practically all of the colors developed in the cells by the Wright's stain are within one sector of this circle or between the blue and the red. This produces a harmony in the colors of the stained blood cells that is pleasing to the eye. It also shows why it is difficult to describe the delicate changes and slight differences in color. The chart expresses only color value; the intensity of color (pink to red, or light blue to deep blue) is not indicated. The points indicated in the center and on the periphery of the circle are the colors at their fullest intensity. The primary colors are indicated by the solid lines and the secondary colors by the broken lines.

5. PLATE I. THE RED CELLS AND THE ERYTHROCYTIC SERIES (Fig. 1)

1. *TERMINOLOGY OF THE NUCLEATED FORMS OF THE ERYTHROCYTIC SERIES.* Before a study of abnormal bloods can be undertaken, the description and terminology of the normal and abnormal forms of red cells must be understood. In the description of the nucleated forms, the characteristics of the nuclear chromatin serve as criteria for classification, since the size of the cell and the color of the cytoplasm are so variable.

All investigators are agreed that the nucleated red cells seen in the blood and in the bone-marrow aspirations in pernicious anemia are abnormally large and that the bone marrow shows an increase in proportion of cells with deeply basophilic cytoplasm. These cells are called " megaloblasts " by many authors. Many of these cells are strikingly atypical, showing clumped or reticular structure of the nucleus, while the cytoplasm is still deeply basophilic. Normally, this type of nuclear structure occurs with a more mature cell, as evidenced by cytoplasm that is less basophilic. There is no evidence that these cells have an origin different from that of normal red cells, although their maturation is abnormal.

Many different names have been applied to the cells of the erythrocytic series. The following list gives the names used in this *Atlas,* in italics, together with the terms employed by other authors: —*stem cell:* haemoblast [224], lymphoidocyte [94, 224], hemocytoblast [56, 139, 185, 301], erythrogone [67]; *proerythroblast* [54, 94, 139, 170, 224, 280]; megaloblast [75, 126], normoblast A [67], pronormoblast [56, 80, 150, 306], rubriblast [48]; *early erythroblast* [54, 75], erythroblast [126], basophilic erythroblast [54, 94, 185, 280], basophilic normoblast [56, 80, 150, 170, 306], early normoblast [139, 301], prorubricyte [48], normoblast B [67]; *late erythroblast* [54, 75]; polychromatic erythroblast [54, 94, 185, 280], polychromatic normoblast [56, 80, 150, 170, 306], pronormoblast [126], intermediate normoblast [139, 301]; *normoblast* [54, 75, 126]: acidophilic erythroblast [54], eosinophilic erythroblast [280], orthochromatic erythroblast [94, 224], orthochromatic normoblast [80, 150, 306], pyknotic normoblast [56], late normoblast [139, 301], normoblast C [67], metarubricyte [48]; *young erythrocyte* (*reticulocyte or polychromatophil*); *adult erythrocyte:* rubricyte [48].

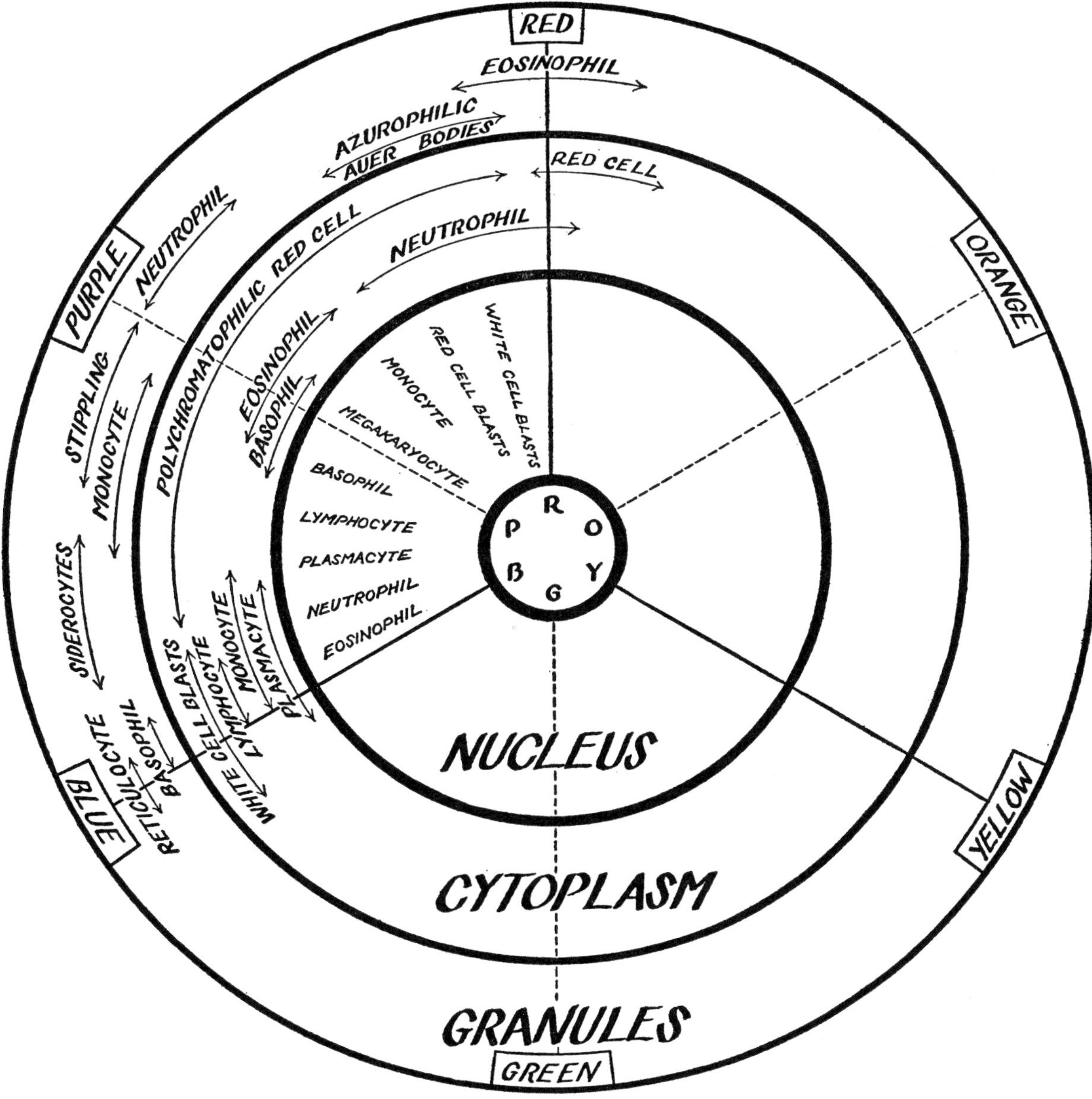

Fig. 2. Graphic representation of the color value of the nucleus, cytoplasm and granules of blood cells stained with Wright's stain.

2. *DESCRIPTION OF NORMAL AND ABNORMAL CELLS OF ERYTHROCYTIC SERIES (PLATE 1).* The cells are described in order from the mature erythrocyte to the least mature form, the proerythroblast. The figures in italics refer to the cells shown in the plate.

(*a*) ERYTHROCYTE (mature red cell, *1*). The diameter of the normal red cell is between 5 and 9 μ with a mean of 7.2 to 7.8 μ in normal individuals. The diameter of the abnormal red cell may vary from 2 to 14 μ. The color of the cell is a yellow-red, owing to staining of hemoglobin. The pale central area results from the thinness of the layer of hemoglobin due to the biconcave shape of the normal red cell. No nucleus or granules are present in the normal red cell.

(*b*) POLYCHROMATOPHILIC ERYTHROCYTE (immature red cell, *2*). This cell is usually larger than the adult cell of the same blood sample. The polychromatophilia is evidenced by the blue-purple color of the cell. No nucleus or granules are normally present, but nucleated red cells may also show polychromasia of the cytoplasm.

Reticulocyte (immature red cell, *7a, 7b, 7c*). This cell is the same stage as the polychromatophilic erythrocyte but is vitally stained with brilliant cresyl blue (pp. 3, 14) so that it can be recognized and counted more easily than polychromatophilic cells. The basophilic material in the cell is precipitated by the cresyl blue as a heavy network of blue substance in the younger forms (*7a*), a moderate amount in the intermediate forms (*7b*), or fine scattered reticulum in the older forms (*7c*). Accordingly, there is a quantitative relation between the amount of reticulum in the cell and the age of the cell [123]. There should be no polychromatophilic cells remaining in a film stained for reticulocytes, since all of the diffuse polychromatophilic material should appear as precipitated reticulum.

(*c*) NORMOBLAST. (*3*). The normoblast may vary in diameter from a normal range of 6 or 7 μ up to 12 to 14 μ in pernicious anemia. The cytoplasm may be acidophilic or polychromatophilic. The nucleus is a small, condensed mass of chromatin, usually deep purple. Very little structure is evident in this compact nucleus. In pathologic conditions the nucleus may be divided into two, three, or more portions (*3e*). In the blood film stained with brilliant cresyl blue, reticulum may be very dense (*3b*) in cells that would show marked polychromatophilia with Wright's stain alone.

(*d*) LATE ERYTHROBLAST (*4*). The erythroblast is larger than the erythrocyte or normoblast. The nuclear chromatin is broken up into segments, sometimes radially arranged like the spokes of a wheel. The cytoplasm at this stage is usually polychromatophilic. For this reason this cell is termed "polychromatophilic erythroblast" by some hematologists.

(*e*) EARLY ERYTHROBLAST (*5*). The chromatin of the nucleus of the early erythroblast is broken up into fine clumps. It is not as granular as in the proerythroblast, but is more finely divided than in the late erythroblast. The cytoplasm is basophilic.

(*f*) PROERYTHROBLAST (*6*). The proerythroblast is the youngest form of the erythrocytic series that can be distinguished from the blasts of the white-cell series. It is usually larger than the normoblast or erythroblast. The cytoplasm is a deep blue (basophilic) with a little more purple than in the other blasts. The nucleus is made up of fine uniformly granular chromatin, is purple in color, and is definitely round in shape. Nucleoli are usually present.

(*g*) STEM CELL. The stem cell is larger than any other blast form (see Plate XV, *8*). The finely granular, purple nucleus is less intense in color than the deeply basophilic cytoplasm. More than one nucleolus may be present in this primitive cell. The stem cell may be seen in the peripheral blood in leukemia in association with other blast forms, or in stem-cell leukemia in which the type of cell is primitive and its series cannot be identified.

(*h*) NUCLEATED RED CELLS IN THE PERIPHERAL BLOOD. Under normal conditions nucleated red cells are found only in the circulating blood of the fetus and newborn infants. Nucleated red cells in the peripheral blood in the adult may occur as a physiologic response to severe anoxia, whether due to anemia from hemorrhage, hemolytic anemia, nutritional or pernicious anemia, or impairment of pulmonary or cardiac functions. The presence of nucleated red cells in the peripheral blood when no evidence of anoxia exists (that is, when the hemoglobin exceeds 10 gm/100 ml of blood and when no cardiac or pulmonary disease is present) should suggest a myelophthisic anemia. Replacement of the bone marrow as a result of carcinoma, lymphoma, leukemia, or fibrosis may cause a myelophthisic anemia.

The pathologic forms of nucleated red cells that are seen in the peripheral blood in the macrocytic anemias associated with Addisonian pernicious anemia, nutritional deficiency, sprue, pernicious anemia of pregnancy, and diphyllobothrium latum infestation are collectively called megaloblasts by many authors. These pathologic forms occur in all stages of the red-cell development, and include abnormal normoblasts (*3a*), abnormal late erythroblasts (*4a*), abnormal early erythroblasts (*5a*), abnormal proerythroblasts (*6a*), and cells showing mitosis (*13*). Many hematologists believe that these pathologic forms of the erythrocytic series show a qualitative change as a result of a deficiency of an essential maturation factor (vitamin B_{12}, folic acid, or citrovorum factor) and do not represent a series of cells of separate origin. These pathologic features are macrocytosis, abnormal reticular structure of the nuclear chromatin, dissynchronism of the maturation of the cytoplasm and the nucleus, and mitosis. Similar abnormalities of size and chromatin structure can also be seen in the circulating granulocytes in these conditions. These changes in red cells, in white cells, and also in megakaryocytes are much more striking in the bone marrow than in the peripheral blood and serve as important diagnostic aids.

The normoblasts in the peripheral blood in iron-deficiency anemia are small and have a scanty amount of basophilic or polychromatophilic cytoplasm. The maturation of the cytoplasm appears to be slower than the maturation of the compact nucleus of the cell. These " iron-deficient " normoblasts are even more striking in the bone marrow.

In hemolytic anemia the nucleated red cells in the peripheral blood are normocytic or macrocytic; they have a normal proportion of the cytoplasmic and nuclear material, and normal structure of nuclear chromatin. Normoblasts with two nuclei (*3e*), with Howell-Jolly bodies (*3d*), with stippling (*3c*), with reticulum (*3b*), and with various other abnormal formations may occur in the hemolytic anemias. These abnormalities are even more striking after splenectomy. In the more severe hemolytic reactions, erythroblasts and rarely proerythroblasts may be present in the peripheral blood.

In the myelophthisic anemias, the nucleated red cells are usually normal in size but may be abortive in form, often having multilobed nuclei or nuclear fragments in the cytoplasm.

(*i*) Stippling, Granules, Nuclear Remnants, and Inclusion Bodies in Red Cells.

Stippled red cells (punctate basophilia). Stippling denotes the presence of round blue-purple granules of variable size scattered throughout the mature, polychromatophilic (*8*), or nucleated (*3c*) red blood cell. Stippled red cells may be seen in films prepared with Wright's stain alone. They are also evident in cresyl blue preparations, but should not be confused with the blue network of the reticulocytes.

Although stippling is a regular characteristic of lead poisoning, it may be seen in normal blood [92], in leukemia, and in practically all the anemias, especially in myelophthisic anemia and in Cooley's anemia and Cooley's trait.

Siderocytes (*10* and *10a*). Nucleated and non-nucleated forms of the red cell with siderotic granules which contain free iron have been termed siderocytes [112]. It is important to recognize and distinguish them from the punctate basophilia of stippled cells and from Howell-Jolly bodies. When stained with Wright's stain, siderotic granules may appear singly as small blue-purple bodies or occur in pairs, or tetrads, near the periphery of the cell. In contrast to the iron contained in hemoglobin, which does not stain, the free iron of the siderotic granule stains greenish blue with the Prussian blue reaction or with acid-iron stain [111, 179]. A dried film of blood is first fixed in methyl alcohol for 10 min and then is dried. It is then immersed for approximately 10 min in a freshly prepared mixture of equal parts of aqueous potassium ferrocyanide (2 gm/100 ml) and aqueous hydrochloric acid (1 percent by volume). The slide is washed, dried, and counterstained with Biebrich scarlet, safranin, or 0.1 percent aqueous basic fuchsin. Finally, the preparation is washed, mounted, and examined with the oil-immersion objective.

Siderocytes have been seen in the embryo and in nucleated red cells of the bone marrow of the adult, but not in the mature erythrocyte of the normal adult [78]. Large numbers may be seen in hemolytic anemia, especially after splenectomy [179, 225].

Howell-Jolly bodies (nuclear remnant, *9*). Howell-Jolly bodies are small (1 to 3 μ), purple-blue, round bodies which may occur singly or in multiples in the red cell. They are stained the same as the nuclei of normoblasts and are considered to be remnants of the nucleus [202]. The cell containing Howell-Jolly bodies (*9*) should be compared with the normoblast with Howell-Jolly bodies (*3d*). In the normoblast, the nucleus apparently is being extruded while two fragments of the nucleus — the size of Howell-Jolly bodies — remain. The diameters of these bodies may vary from that of a small nucleus down to 0.5 μ. Howell-Jolly bodies are seen in severe anemias such as pernicious anemia, Cooley's anemia, erythroblastosis, and sickle-cell anemia. They are increased in the blood of normal persons following splenectomy [168], and appear to be found characteristically in patients with atrophy of the spleen [28] in a variety of conditions including sprue and nontropical sprue.

Cabot ring forms (*14*). Red cells in certain anemias occasionally show a delicate violet threadlike structure in the form of a ring or twisted ring or figure of eight. Cabot [35] originally described these structures and considered them to be remnants of the nuclear membrane. Schleicher [255], however, has presented evidence that the rings are artifacts due to formation of denatured protein. The rare occurrence of these rings has made study of them difficult.

Refractive granule of red blood cell (*11*). A refractive body about 0.5 μ in diameter occurring in less than 1 percent of normal red cells was described by Isaacs [136]. This granule, which occurs singly, appears black in one focal plane of the microscope and clear and colorless (refractive) in another. It does not take any ordinary stains and is of unknown origin and composition. The occurrence of granules is similar to that of the reticulocytes, but red cells containing granules are considered to represent a more mature, or intermediate, stage between the reticulocyte and the mature erythrocyte.

Heinz-Ehrlich bodies (refractive bodies, *12*). Refractive bodies in red cells, described by Heinz [125] and by Ehrlich [84], are seen in wet preparations and are not stained by Romanowsky stains. They appear in the red cells as round refractile inclusion bodies with Brownian movement, varying in diameter from 0.5 to 1 μ. They appear to be newly formed particles containing protein (of unknown origin) and occur in the course of irreversible injury to the red cell by certain toxic agents [95, 298]. In contrast to the refractive granule of Isaacs, the Heinz-Ehrlich bodies are associated with hemolytic anemias from such compounds as phenylhydrazine, erythrol tetranitrate, and the sulfonamides. An extensive study of other compounds that produce Heinz-Ehrlich bodies has been made by Fertman and Fertman [96]. They can be stained vitally by employing a half-saturated solution of methyl violet or crystal violet in saline [299]. One drop of this solution and one drop of blood are placed on a slide, covered with a coverglass, and observed under high magnification (× 1000). The granules appear as blue-violet particles often near the periphery of the cell.

(*j*) Abnormal Shapes of Red Cells. The terms *anisocytosis* (abnormal variation in size) and *poikilocytosis* (abnormal variation in shape) have been used too loosely in describing the red cells in pathologic conditions. Instead of using these terms, it is of greater diagnostic value to observe and describe the particular abnormal forms and associate them with a specific disease entity. For example, the presence of polychromatophilic macrocytes usually means active regeneration of blood, which may be due to hemolytic anemia, acute blood loss, or response to therapy. The presence of definite sickled forms (*24*) is diagnostic of the sickle-cell phenomenon, but the phenomenon should be confirmed by a specific test.

Spheroidal red cells (spherocytes, *19*). The spheroidal red cell is a small deeply stained cell without central pallor, in which the hemoglobin appears increased. Since the volume of the spherocyte is approximately normal but its diameter is less than normal, it is apparent, geometrically, that its thickness is increased. Microscopically, the cells appear hyperchromic not only because of this increased thickness but also because of their increased corpuscular hemoglobin concentration (MCHC). Spheroidal red cells have increased osmotic and mechanical fragility, and they occur in congenital hemolytic jaundice (hereditary spherocytosis), in other hemolytic anemias such as acquired hemolytic anemia, following thermal burns [260], and in certain drug intoxications [87].

Oval cells (elliptic cells). Oval macrocytes (*16*) are characteristic cells that are usually seen in the blood film of untreated pernicious anemia. However, oval cells (*17*) that are approximately normal in size are occasionally seen in increased numbers in the peripheral blood as an inherited Mendelian dominant characteristic [279]. A comprehensive study of 86 cases in three interrelated families was made by Wyandt, Bancroft, and Winship [313]. Only one of these cases showed striking anemia. This patient undoubtedly had the oval-cell characteristic in the homozygous state while the other members had the factor as a heterozygote. Lipton [176] has reported a patient who was homozygous for the elliptocytic trait and had a severe anemia. Some individuals with oval cells have had by coincidence other blood dyscrasias, such as pernicious anemia, leukemia, and hemolytic jaundice. Oval cells do not sickle, although some cases of ovalocytosis reported in the literature have been confused with sickle-cell anemia.

Pencil forms (*18*). The pencil form of red cells, which may be confused with the oval cells, is thinner in proportion to its length than the oval cell. Pencil forms are usually hypochromic and are characteristically found in hypochromic anemia, Cooley's anemia, and Cooley's trait.

Sickle cells (*24*). Sickled forms of red cells are sometimes, but not always, seen in the film of peripheral blood of a patient with sickle-cell anemia. These may take the forms shown in Plate I (*24*) or they may have more rounded ends. Those with rounded ends are permanently (irreversibly) sickled forms [259]. Those with pointed ends or filaments, seen in freshly sickled preparations, may not be evident in the untreated film of peripheral blood. (See Plate VI.)

Target cells (*26*). The " target " cell has created more interest and been described by more names (Mexican hat, button form, bull's-eye) than it deserves. Because of its unique arrangement of hemoglobin, it looks like a target, that is, there is a central area of hemoglobin (bull's-eye), surrounded by a clear ring without pigment, outside of which is the pigmented border of the cell. These cells are thin hypochromic cells which show an increased resistance to hemolysis in hypotonic solutions of sodium chloride [14, 113]. They are seen in increased numbers in severe hypochromic anemia, sickle-cell anemia, Cooley's anemia and trait, liver disease, and in patients with hemoglobin C disease, and are often increased in number following splenectomy [268]. Target cells may be produced in vitro by suspending normal red cells in plasma or serum, rendered hypertonic either by addition of chemicals or by evaporation [293]. It is possible to see target cells in certain areas of a film of normal blood; their presence, however, may be due to abnormal drying of the film and should not be considered typical of the blood picture unless it is seen throughout the film.

Lunar forms (*20*). Lunar or half-moon forms have been seen in acute hemolytic anemia (Plate VII). " Shadows " or ghosts of erythrocytes, thin veils of membrane, and " crescent bodies " — colorless veillike disks 40 to 50 μ in diameter with pink crescents in the margin — are found only rarely as a result of hemolysis [306].

Crenated red cells (*21*). Red cells are sometimes distorted owing to changes in surface. These round cells have numerous regularly spaced points or spicules on the surface. Such cells frequently occur in groups in certain areas of the film.

Burr cell (*22*). A poikilocyte with one to several large spiny projections on its periphery has been called a " burr " cell because of its resemblance to a burr. This cell usually occurs singly and not in groups as do crenated cells. Schwartz *et al.* [257] found an increase of these cells in uremia, carcinoma of the stomach, and bleeding peptic ulcer.

Acanthrocyte (*23*). The acanthrocyte is a deformed red cell that has numerous irregularly spaced and irregularly shaped pseudopods on its periphery, giving the appearance of thorns [265].

These cells were originally reported by Bassen and Kornzweig [15] in a case of atypical retinitis pigmentosa.

Irregular form (poikilocytes, *25, 27*). A variety of terms — such as pear-shaped, tailed, or bizarre forms — are used to describe the irregular forms of cells seen in certain of the red-cell diseases. It is unknown by what mechanism these forms arise, whether fragmentation of red cells, budding of the cytoplasm to produce daughter cells, or defective formation of cells [51, 77, 248]. Small round particles containing hemoglobin were called schistocytes by Ehrlich [86]. It is known that fission of the red cells occurs as a result of heating [118, 137]. Tiny microcytes are often seen in the blood in hypochromic anemia, pernicious anemia, and Cooley's anemia. The presence of a variety of these shapes and of microcytes is a characteristic feature and aids in the diagnosis of Cooley's anemia.

3. *COUNTING RETICULOCYTES.* In either a dry or a wet preparation, the number of reticulocytes is determined by counting a total of 1000 red cells. All red cells, including nucleated forms, that contain reticulum are counted as reticulocytes. The results are usually expressed as a percentage of the total number of red cells; or the absolute number of reticulocytes per unit volume may be calculated from the red-cell count. Because of the large number of cells in an oil-immersion field, it is helpful to cut down the area by inserting, in one ocular of the microscope, a mask that has a central hole 3 to 5 mm in diameter. Different areas where the film is thin and the cells are separated, well stained, and easily identified should be selected for counting.

Counterstaining the vitally stained preparation with Wright's stain, although not essential, gives a sharp contrast between the blue of the reticulum and the red of the cell. No polychromatophilic cells should be present if the film is sufficiently stained with brilliant cresyl blue. A film that is poorly stained should be discarded. Precipitated stain is often confused with reticulum, but may be recognized because it occurs outside as well as on the red cells; it may be avoided by thorough washing after staining and frequent filtering of the cresyl blue and Wright's stain. Platelets superimposed on red cells may also be confused with reticulum. Reticulum is definitely blue, whereas the granules of platelets are purple. The amount of reticulum varies from a dense network of disconnected but multiple blue particles to one or two small particles. Any cell containing material recognizable as reticulum is included in the reticulocyte count.

The normal values for reticulocytes vary slightly with the method employed, but are usually in the range of 0.5 to 1.5 percent. The number of reticulocytes should be as great as, or greater than, the number of polychromatophilic cells seen in a smear taken simultaneously but stained only with Wright's stain.

4. *DETERMINATION OF VARIATION FROM THE NORMAL IN SIZE, SHAPE, AND HEMOGLOBIN CONTENT OF RED CELLS.* A careful study of the blood film will show the variation from normal of the morphologic characteristics of the red cells in respect to size, shape, and hemoglobin content. When these abnormalities are striking there is little difficulty in classifying the cells as macrocytic, normocytic, or microcytic, and as normochromic or hypochromic. When the changes are slight, it is necessary to compare the cells with those of a normal individual.

(*a*) Comparison with a Film of Normal Blood. It is always possible to have at hand a normal film that may be interchanged with the abnormal film and observed under the microscope for comparison with an unknown film. For a direct comparison with a normal film a satisfactory preparation of the unknown blood stained with Wright's stain is mounted on a glass slide with the blood film up. A film of normal blood on a coverglass, also stained with Wright's stain, is then mounted with immersion oil, stained side down, on top of the unknown film. The two films are then face to face and can be focused upon alternately and quickly, using the oil-immersion objective, so that the unknown and normal red cells can be compared for size, shape, and hemoglobin content. The films are of necessity placed in this manner, because in any other combination they are separated by too great a distance to permit focusing with the oil-immersion lens on the lower film.

(*b*) Determination of Mean Cell Volume

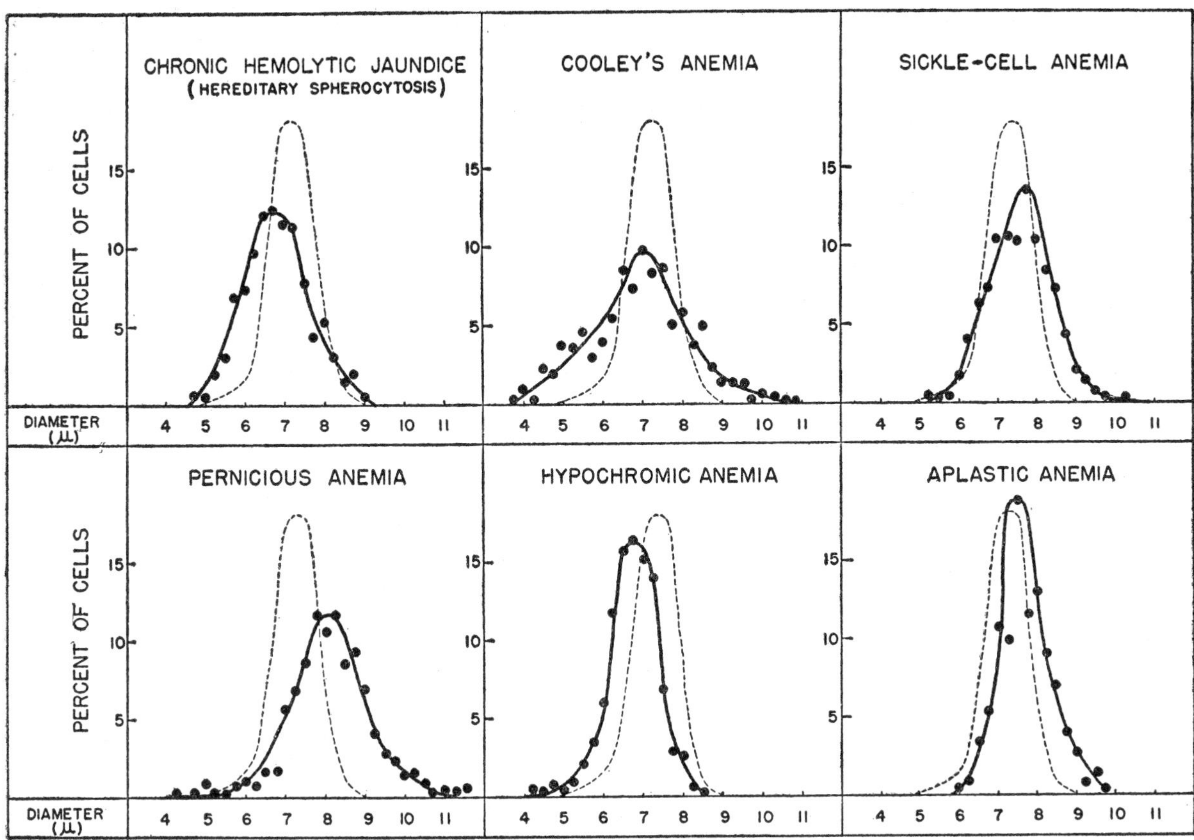

FIG. 3. Typical curves of the frequency distribution of red-cell diameters in six examples of anemia compared in each instance to a curve (dotted line) derived from ten normal subjects (see Table 1).

TABLE 1. DATA FOR THE FREQUENCY-DISTRIBUTION CURVES OF RED-CELL DIAMETERS SHOWN IN FIG. 3 *

Diagnosis	Red-cell count (10^6/mm^3)	Hemoglobin (gm/100 ml)	Hematocrit (percent)	Mean corpuscular volume, MCV (μ^3)	Mean corpuscular hemoglobin concentration, MCHC †	Mean cell diameter, MCD (μ)	Standard deviation of diameter, σ	Coefficient of variation of diameter (percent)	Mean cell thickness, MCT (μ)
	Mean values for 10 normal individuals								
Normal subjects	4.81	14.7	44.7	93	33	7.2	0.50	7.0	2.3
	Chronic hemolytic anemias, characterized by hereditary defects of the red cells								
Congenital (chronic) hemolytic jaundice	3.34	10.0	29.7	89	34	6.83	0.80	11.8	2.43
Cooley's anemia	3.82	7.2	27.7	73	26	6.92	1.27	19.8	1.93
Sickle-cell anemia	3.46	7.8	24.8	72	31	7.61	0.84	10.5	1.65
	Anemias due to decreased production of red cells								
Pernicious anemia	1.16	4.2	14.5	125	29	8.10	1.01	12.5	2.43
Hypochromic anemia	2.72	4.2	16.7	61	25	6.70	0.64	9.5	1.74
Aplastic anemia	1.48	6.0	16.1	109	37	7.7	0.71	9.2	2.34

* The indices (mean corpuscular volume, mean corpuscular hemoglobin concentration, and mean corpuscular hemoglobin) were calculated according to Wintrobe [305]. The mean cell diameter was measured according to the method of Price-Jones [234], standard deviation and coefficient of variation also being determined. The mean thickness of the cells was calculated from this mean volume and mean diameter according to the method of von Boros [27], on the assumption that the red cell is a right circular cylinder of known volume and diameter.

† Grams of hemoglobin per 100 ml of packed red cells.

AND HEMOGLOBIN BY THE WINTROBE METHOD [305]. Any blood that shows significant variation from the normal should have a red-cell count, hemoglobin, and hematocrit with determination of the red-cell indices of Wintrobe (MCV, MCHC, MCH). These indices give the mean values for volume and hemoglobin concentration, but do not give any estimate of the degree of variation, which is evaluated by visual examination of the film or by the Price-Jones method discussed in the next paragraph. These values should be compared and correlated with those observed in the films for size and hemoglobin concentration.

(*c*) MEAN DIAMETER AND VARIATION OF DIAMETER AND THICKNESS OF RED CELL. The mean size and variation in size of red cells can be determined, from measurement of the cell diameters, by the method of Price-Jones [234]. The data can be shown graphically as a distribution curve, as in Fig. 3, or analyzed statistically by determining the frequency of occurrence of diameters in each group (using differences of $\frac{1}{4}$ μ). The mean cell diameter (MCD), the standard deviation of the diameter from the mean, and the coefficient of variation are determined. The standard deviation of the diameters of a population of red cells expresses quantitatively the degree of variation from the mean diameter. Since the absolute values for the mean diameter vary in different conditions, the more useful statistical measure for comparison of results is the coefficient of variation from the mean diameter, which is expressed in percent (Table 1).

As shown in Fig. 3, three hereditary anemias are characterized by abnormalities of the geometry of the red cells. In congenital hemolytic jaundice, the mean cell diameter is decreased, so that the red cells appear microcytic on the blood film. However, the mean cell volume (MCV) is normal or slightly increased, so that the mean cell thickness (MCT) is abnormally increased and the cells are more spheroidal than normal, a fact that renders them more susceptible to osmotic and mechanical hemolysis [27, 40, 113]. In sickle-cell anemia the mean diameter is increased, so that the red cells appear macrocytic on the blood film. However, the mean cell volume is not increased, but normal or slightly decreased, so the thickness is decreased. The increased flatness of these cells renders them less susceptible to osmotic hemolysis. In Cooley's anemia, which is usually microcytic, the coefficient of variation of the diameters is greater than in any other anemia and the microcytes predominate over the macrocytes.

In pernicious anemia, the coefficient of variation is also large, greater than in any other macrocytic anemia [61]. In many instances of aplastic anemia, the cells may be macrocytic, but the distribution of the diameters is approximately normal. In hypochromic anemia, the variation in diameter of the red cells is not so marked as in Cooley's anemia, although the cells show an increasing degree of microcytosis and variation in diameter as the iron deficiency increases.

6. PLATE II. THE WHITE CELLS

1. *INTRODUCTION.* The white blood cells are divided into five separate series, namely, granulocytic, lymphocytic, plasmacytic, monocytic, and histiocytic [53]. The maturation and nuclear structure of the cells in each of the first four of these series are illustrated diagrammatically in Figs. 4, 5, 6, and 7. The structure of histiocytic cells is shown in Fig. 8. It is not always essential, when a differential count is made, to subdivide each series into as many stages as are shown in the figures, but it is necessary to recognize these stages in order to understand the degree of maturity of each cell. In general, the more immature the cells, the more serious is the prognosis in diseases of the blood and in physiologic responses. Typical cells representing each stage are described. It is not always possible to classify the cells since there are many intermediate stages, and abortive and abnormal forms. Sometimes the nucleus develops faster than the cytoplasm and sometimes the cytoplasm is more mature than would be expected with the structure of the nu-

cleus. Typical cells seen in normal blood are shown in Plate II.

2. *GRANULOCYTIC SERIES* (Fig. 4 and Plates II, X, and XI).

(*a*) NEUTROPHIL (polymorphonuclear neutrophil, granulocyte; Plate II, *3*, *3a*). The neutrophil has a diameter of approximately 10 to 15 μ. The nucleus shows two or more distinct lobes connected by bands or threads of chromatin, and is made up of coarse condensed masses of purple-staining chromatin. The cytoplasm is pink to lilac. The granules, if present, are fine and have the color of the nucleus (neutrophilic).

Abnormal forms. Hypersegmented or multilobed neutrophils are found in untreated pernicious anemia, although they may occur in other conditions. Round or oval basophilic areas in the cytoplasm, known as Döhle bodies, may be seen in certain infections. In certain other infections, toxic granules which appear as blue-black, coarse granules may occur in the cytoplasm. Occasionally these granules are mistaken for those of the basophil.

(*b*) EOSINOPHIL. The eosinophils are a little larger than neutrophils. This is especially true when the cells are poured forth in large numbers, as in certain infestations, such as trichiniasis, or other pathologic states. The nucleus is usually bilobed or a band form (Plate II, *5a*, *5b*). The cytoplasm is usually lilac to blue, but may be difficult to see because of the large number of granules. The granules are much larger than those seen in the neutrophil or in any other cell. They are a bright orange-red in color and sharply defined or round in outline. They often appear over the nucleus, as well as free in the cytoplasm.

(*c*) BASOPHIL. Basophils (Plate II, *6a*, *6b*) are usually a little smaller than the mature neutrophil. The nucleus is lobulated as in the neutrophil. The cytoplasm is usually lilac to blue. Large distinct blue granules are generally scattered throughout the cell and may be so numerous as to obscure the structure of the nucleus.

(*d*) YOUNG GRANULOCYTE OR BAND FORM (stab, young form; Plate II, *4*). The band forms of the neutrophil are immature cells which are often slightly larger than the mature forms with the corresponding granulation. There may also be band forms of the eosinophil and basophil. The nucleus of the cell is not segmented. The cytoplasm is the color of the corresponding adult cell. The granules are the same as those of the adult cell of the series, being fine purple granules in the young neutrophil, large blue granules in the young basophil (Plate II, *6a*), and red-orange granules in the eosinophilic cell. The band form is the predominating cell in Pelger's anomaly [133].

(*e*) METAMYELOCYTE. The nucleus is round, indented, or kidney-shaped, and the clumps of chromatin are not so deeply stained as in the older cells. The cytoplasm and granules are similar to those of the corresponding adult cell.

(*f*) MYELOCYTE C (late myelocyte). The nucleus is round and quite distinct in outline. The smooth structure of the nucleus is contrasted with the clumped chromatin of the more mature forms. The cytoplasm is more basophilic than in the metamyelocytes or later forms. Granules may be neutrophilic, eosinophilic, or basophilic, and, if present, are in the cytoplasm and are *not* seen over the nucleus.

(*g*) MYELOCYTE B. This cell is usually much larger than the more mature cells of this series (12 to 18 μ). The nucleus, which may be round or oval, is less sharply defined than in any other cell. The chromatin structure is rather homogeneous. The cytoplasm is more basophilic than in the older cells. The granules are scattered throughout the entire cytoplasm and *cover* the nucleus. Often the contour of the nucleus is obscured by the granules. The granules may be neutrophilic, eosinophilic, or basophilic (or specific). The eosinophilic and basophilic granules are larger than the neutrophilic granules, but smaller than the corresponding type of granule in the older cells. (This is the earliest stage in which specific granulation appears.)

(*h*) MYELOCYTE A (promyelocyte). The nucleus is a deep red-purple, with a fine granular structure. Nucleoli may or may not be present. A nucleolus is a small, round, sharply defined area in the nucleus that takes a light-blue stain. The cytoplasm is a deep blue. A few scattered red-purple or azurophilic granules appear. These granules are usually nonspecific, since differentiation into neutrophilic, eosinophilic, and basophilic

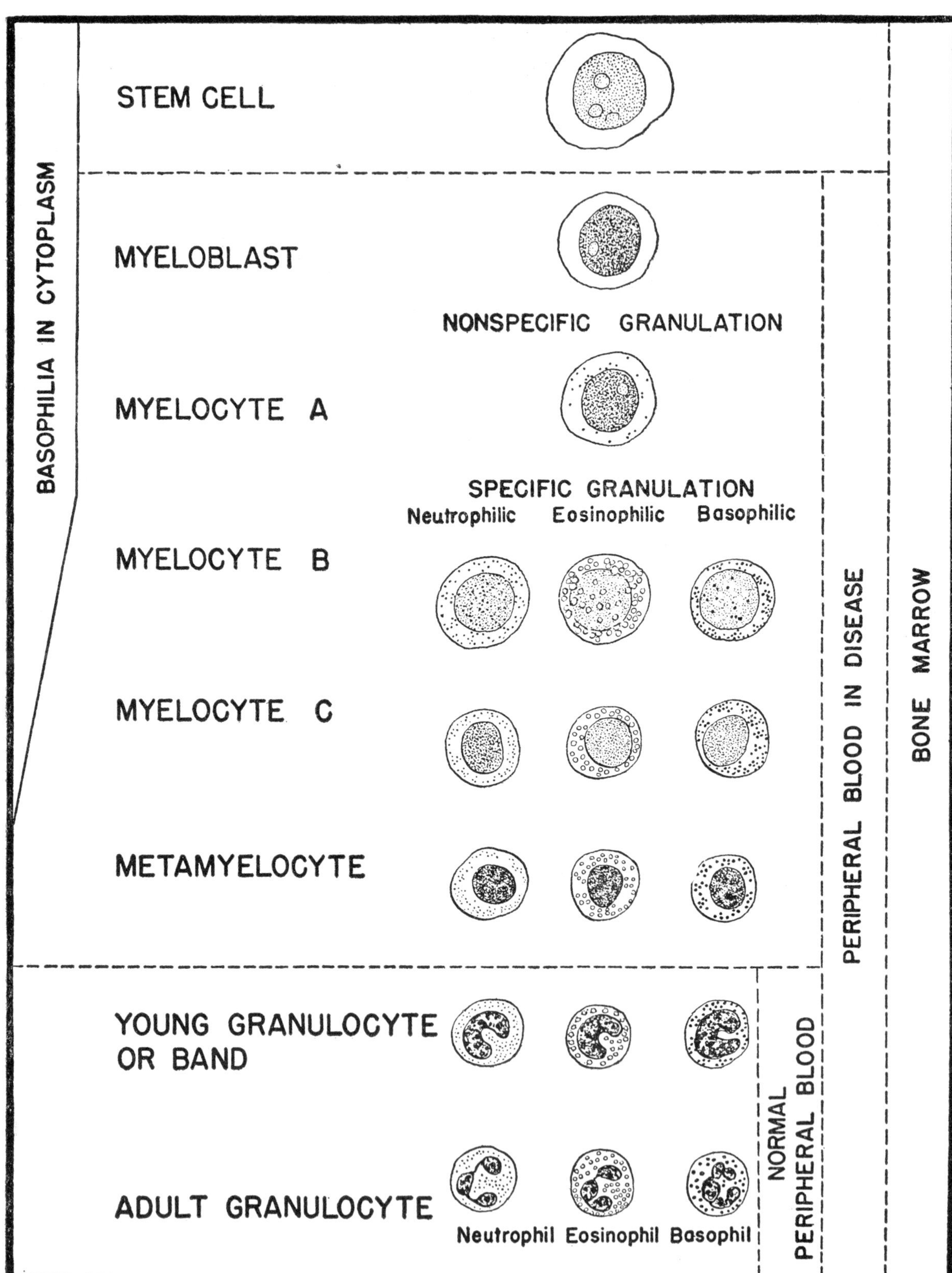

FIG. 4. Diagram of the maturation of the granulocytic series.

granules takes place at a more mature stage (myelocyte B).

(*i*) Myeloblast. The nucleus is red-purple with a finely granular or homogeneous chromatin structure. There are usually one to three nucleoli present in the form of round blue areas. The intensity of color of the nucleus is often less than that of the cytoplasm. The cytoplasm is intensely basophilic. No granules are present. It may be impossible to distinguish the myeloblast from other blast forms.

(*j*) Stem Cell (same as described above, p. 10).

3. *LYMPHOCYTIC SERIES* (Fig. 5 and Plates II, XIV, and XVI).

(*a*) Small Lymphocyte (Plate II, *7*). The small, adult lymphocyte is the smallest white cell (7 to 10 μ). The nucleus is deep purple and usually about the size of the red cell. The round nucleus is made up of masses of chromatin, so that no distinctive internal structure is seen. The periphery of the nucleus is usually defined rather sharply. The cytoplasm forms a narrow rim around the nucleus. This cytoplasm should be a clear light blue, but often in thick or heavily stained smears the color is rather dark. Occasionally red-purple granules and, more rarely, blue granules are present in the cytoplasm. These granules, however, are few, distinct, and scattered, and should not be confused with the finer granules of the monocyte.

(*b*) Large Lymphocyte (Plate II, *8*). The large lymphocyte varies in diameter from 10 to 18 μ and may be as large as a monocyte. The nucleus is usually somewhat larger than in the small lymphocyte and is often irregular in shape; the chromatin masses are not clumped quite as much as in the small lymphocytes and may sometimes have a smooth appearance. The cytoplasm is a clear light blue and is much greater in proportion to the nucleus than in the small lymphocyte. Occasionally red-purple granules may be scattered through the cytoplasm.

(*c*) Young Lymphocyte. The young lymphocyte occurs occasionally in normal bloods, and frequently in children's blood and in the blood in infectious states. This cell is the size of the large lymphocyte, but the nucleus fills a greater proportion of the cell. Chromatin masses of the nucleus are not so condensed as in the older forms, but do not resemble the fine structure of a blast form. A deep-blue basophilic cytoplasm is characteristic of these young cells. No granules are present.

(*d*) Lymphoblast. The red-purple nucleus is made up of finely granular chromatin, with or without nucleoli, as in other blasts. The cytoplasm of the cell is deeply basophilic, as is characteristic of other blast forms. Sometimes there is a clear perinuclear area in the cytoplasm. Occasionally blasts appear with almost no cytoplasm but containing the characteristic nucleus. Granules are absent. The lymphoblast may be indistinguishable from other blast forms.

(*e*) Stem Cell (same as described above, p. 10).

(*f*) Atypical Lymphocytes (Plate XVI). Among the abnormal cells of the lymphocytic series, those seen in infectious mononucleosis are of especial interest. These cells vary markedly in their characteristics but three definite types may be recognized. These abnormal forms may be seen in normal blood in small numbers, but are seen in increased numbers in infectious mononucleosis, infectious hepatitis, chicken pox, and serum sickness.

One variety of atypical lymphocyte may be seen that is larger than the large lymphocyte and usually of irregular shape (appearing to have many sides). The irregular periphery gives the appearance of a distorted cell, and the presence of so many of these irregularities of outline suggests that these cells are abnormally fragile. The cytoplasm is a hyaline blue without granules. The intensity of blue may be increased along the margin of the cell as if the cytoplasm were thicker or condensed along the edge. The irregular nucleus is often more reticular and more wavy than that of the normal lymphocyte, and for this reason may be confused with the monocyte.

A second variety of atypical lymphocyte includes cells of large size and irregular shape similar to the first variety. The chief characteristic of the second variety is the deep muddy-blue color of the cytoplasm. Although this basophilic cytoplasm is typical of immature cells or blast forms, the nuclear structure is quite mature in appearance, the nuclear chromatin occurring in wavy masses. Granules are usually absent.

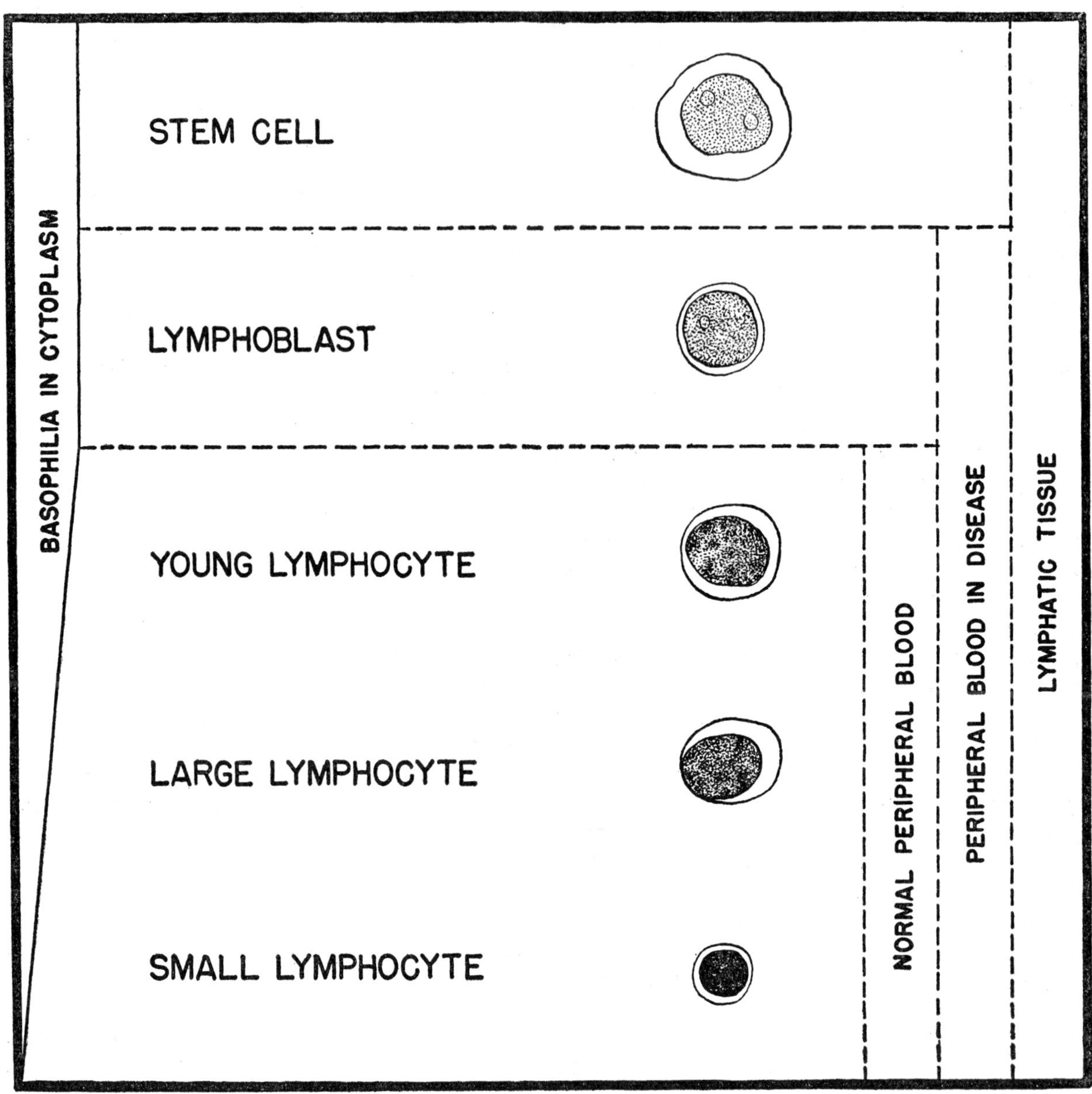

Fig. 5. Diagram of the maturation of the lymphocytic series.

In a third variety of atypical lymphocyte, the cytoplasm is vacuolated in variable degree. If the vacuolation is marked, it may give a " foamy " appearance. The cytoplasm may be light blue or a very deep blue.

4. *PLASMACYTIC SERIES* (Fig. 6 and Plate XV).

(*a*) Plasma Cell (plasmacyte). The nucleus of the plasma cell (plasmacyte) has a very characteristic coarse, deeply stained, clumped chromatin structure. This nucleus is usually eccentrically placed in an oval or elongated cell. The cytoplasm is a deep green-blue with a spongy appearance. There are often vacuoles in the cytoplasm. Globules or clear areas in the cytoplasm taking an acid stain are called Russell bodies. These may occur singly or in groups, or they may rupture to make a larger, irregular, acidophilic

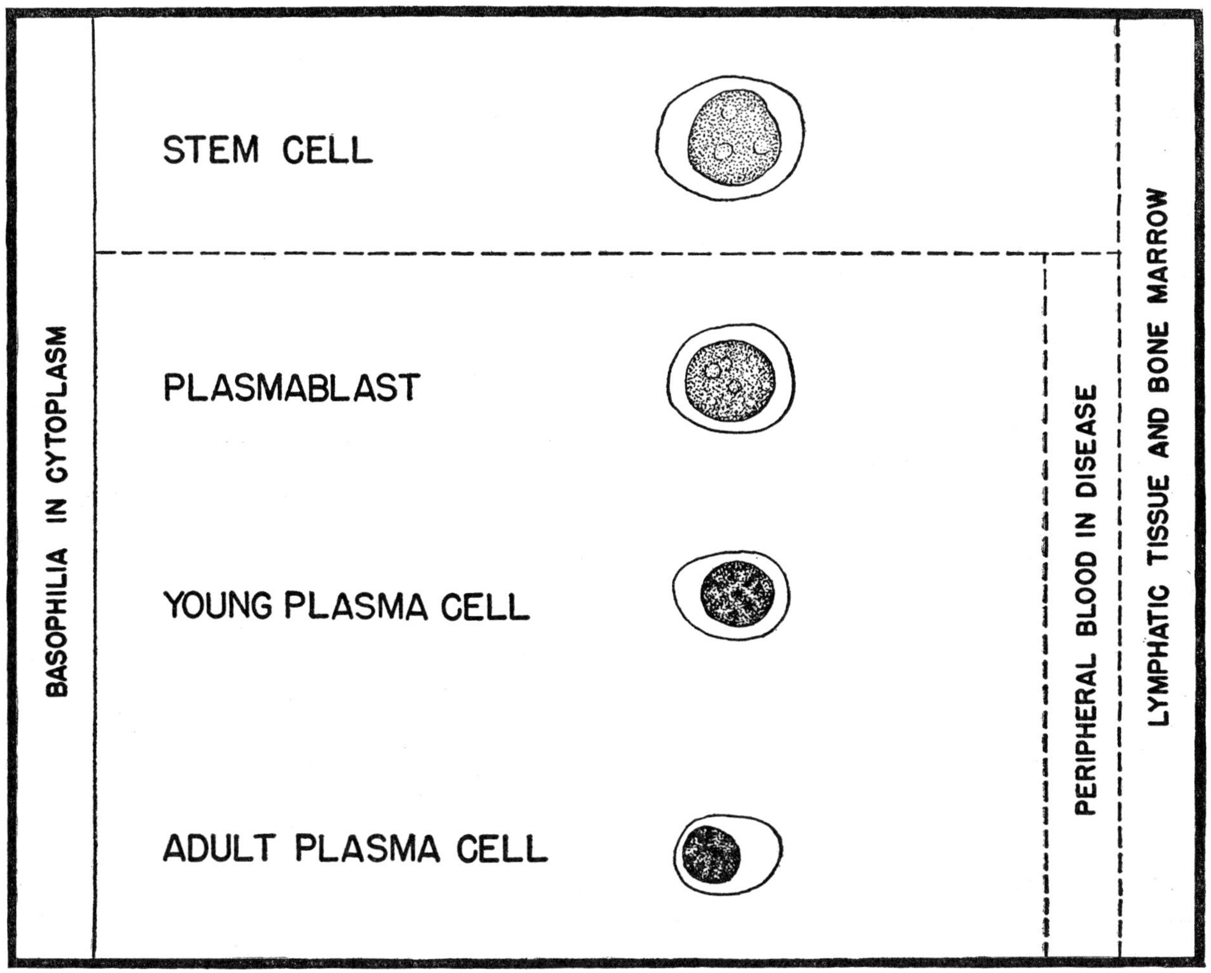

FIG. 6. Diagram of the maturation of the plasmacytic series.

area, often seen around the edge of plasma cells. The edge of the cytoplasm may be very ragged or fringed. Granules are rare in the plasma cell, but basophilic granules may occur. Large basophilic granules which appear following treatment with stilbamidine are called inclusion bodies.

(*b*) YOUNG PLASMA CELL. The young plasma cell is usually larger than the adult plasma cell and has been described as the " multiple myeloma " cell. The nucleus has a finer structure than that of the adult cell, the chromatin often occurring in smaller clumps, sometimes granular. The nucleus is not necessarily eccentric in position. The color of the cytoplasm is the same green-blue as the adult cell, but may be more intense. The spongy appearance may be evident and vacuoles may be present.

(*c*) PLASMABLAST. The nucleus has a fine granular structure that is typical of all blasts. One or more large, sharply defined nucleoli are present. The cytoplasm has the green-blue color that is characteristic of this series of cells. Vacuoles may be present. The plasmablast may not be distinguishable from other blast forms in some instances.

(*d*) STEM CELL (same as described above, p. 10).

(*e*) ABNORMAL FORMS. The presence of large, irregular plasma cells with characteristic nuclei, but with abundant cytoplasm and indefinite ragged peripheries, sometimes with streamers of cytoplasm, may be of significance and not artifactitious. Although the eccentric nucleus is characteristic, it should be recognized that in pathologic conditions there are abortive forms and this is, therefore, not an essential criterion. Although the diameter of these cells varies from 10 to 20 μ, the younger forms are larger than the adult cell. In pathologic conditions, such as plasmocytoma, there are often abnormally large forms, and sometimes cells with more than one nucleus.

(*f*) Comparison of Plasma Cells with Other Cells. The color of the cytoplasm in the plasmacytic series is a characteristic muddy green-blue, the younger forms being a deeper, more intense blue. This blue is much deeper than that seen in the cytoplasm of any lymphocyte and more of a green-blue than that seen in other blast forms. The cytoplasm of the plasmacytic series is sometimes confused with that of the monocyte, but lacks the granules of the monocyte and is a much deeper blue and more opaque in appearance.

5. *MONOCYTIC SERIES* (Fig. 7 and Plate XII).

(*a*) Monocyte (Plate II, *9*). The monocyte is larger than most of the other cells that are found in the normal peripheral blood (13 to 20 μ). The nucleus is indented or lobulated, often presenting a folded appearance. The structure of the nucleus is looser than that of any of the other cells, as if it were made up of a network of chromatin. Because of this lacy structure, the nucleus appears to be stained lighter purple than the nuclei of other cells. The cytoplasm is a gray-blue, in contrast to the clear light blue of the lymphocytes. The granulation varies in different cases. The monocyte usually contains fine neutrophilic granules, although in some cells red-purple granules are scattered throughout the cytoplasm. The amount of granulation varies from none to a dense stippling of fine granules.

(*b*) Young Monocyte (Plate II, *10*). The nucleus in the young monocyte is round, but the same lacy folded type of nucleus is seen as is present in the adult monocyte. The cytoplasm is the same gray-blue as in the adult form. This cell should be compared with the adult cell in a given smear to differentiate the cell from the lymphocyte or the metamyelocyte. The granules are the same as in the adult cell.

(*c*) Monoblast. The nucleus of the monoblast is much finer in structure than in the older cells of the series, although the contour may be irregular, and it may have a certain folded appearance characteristic of the adult cell. Although the chromatin is finely granular, it is more lacy than in the other types of blasts. Nucleoli are usually present. The cytoplasm is a deep blue, showing more gray-blue than in the myeloblast or lymphoblast. There may be red-purple granules in this blast form, even in the presence of nucleoli. Auer bodies, which appear as short red rods or splinters, are frequently present in the monoblast.

(*d*) Stem Cell (same as described above, p. 10).

6. *HISTIOCYTIC SERIES* (Fig. 8 and Plate XIII). The histiocyte, as seen in the peripheral blood and bone marrow, represents a series of cells that are derived from the reticulo-endothelial tissue throughout the body and can be differentiated from other series of white cells, such as the monocytic.

Histiocytes have been referred to by many terms, such as large mononuclear leukocytes; macrophages of Metchnikoff, 1892; endothelial leukocyte of Mallory, 1898; adventitial cells of Marchand, 1898; clasmatocyte of Ranvier, 1900, and of Sabin, Doan, and Cunningham, 1923–24; histiocyte of Aschoff and Kiyono, 1913; endothelial phagocyte of Foot, 1925; and monocyte by many investigators in recent years [98, 251, 252]. Much experimental and clinical work on histiocytes is difficult to interpret because the cells were classified as monocytes.

Histiocytes may be present in the peripheral-blood film of normal individuals.

The appearance of histiocytes varies greatly in the same blood film, in different samples from the same individual, and in samples from different individuals under pathologic conditions. This variation in the type of cell seen may be related to the tissue from which the cells arise (spleen or lymph nodes) and to the process for which they are elaborated. In histiocytic leukemia, the histiocytes, which may be markedly increased, are probably the result of abnormal growth of a particular cell type with proliferation in the peripheral blood as well as tissues. No maturation cycle has been established for the histiocytic series. Nucleoli may be present in cells that do not show basophilic cytoplasm, while some of the most basophilic cells may lack nucleoli.

Histiocytes are larger than the cells of the erythrocytic or white-cell series and usually are markedly irregular in shape. A few recognized types of histiocytes are described since no single description is adequate.

(*a*) Histiocyte — Amoeboid Form. The amoeboid form of histiocyte is larger than the monocyte or lymphocyte, but is often confused with them (Plate XII, *5*). The nucleus has a definite but delicate membrane, and is lighter in color than that of the lymphocyte or monocyte. The nucleus may appear as a loose network or as a structure resembling a honeycomb. There may be one or more small blue nucleoli. The abundant cytoplasm is a pale gray-blue so delicate that the cell membrane is quite difficult to discern. The irregular shape of the cell resembles an amoeba, pseudopods of cytoplasm being very characteristic. In some cells there appears to be endoplasm containing fine granules, surrounded by a clear, pale-blue ectoplasm. The granules, if present, are fine and red-purple in color. Irregular black particles or cellular debris may be present.

(*b*) Histiocyte — Phagocytic Form. The phagocytic histiocyte is very large (15 to 80 μ) and irregular in shape. The nucleus is light purple and reticular, sometimes with one or two nucleoli. The cytoplasm is characterized by delicate lav-

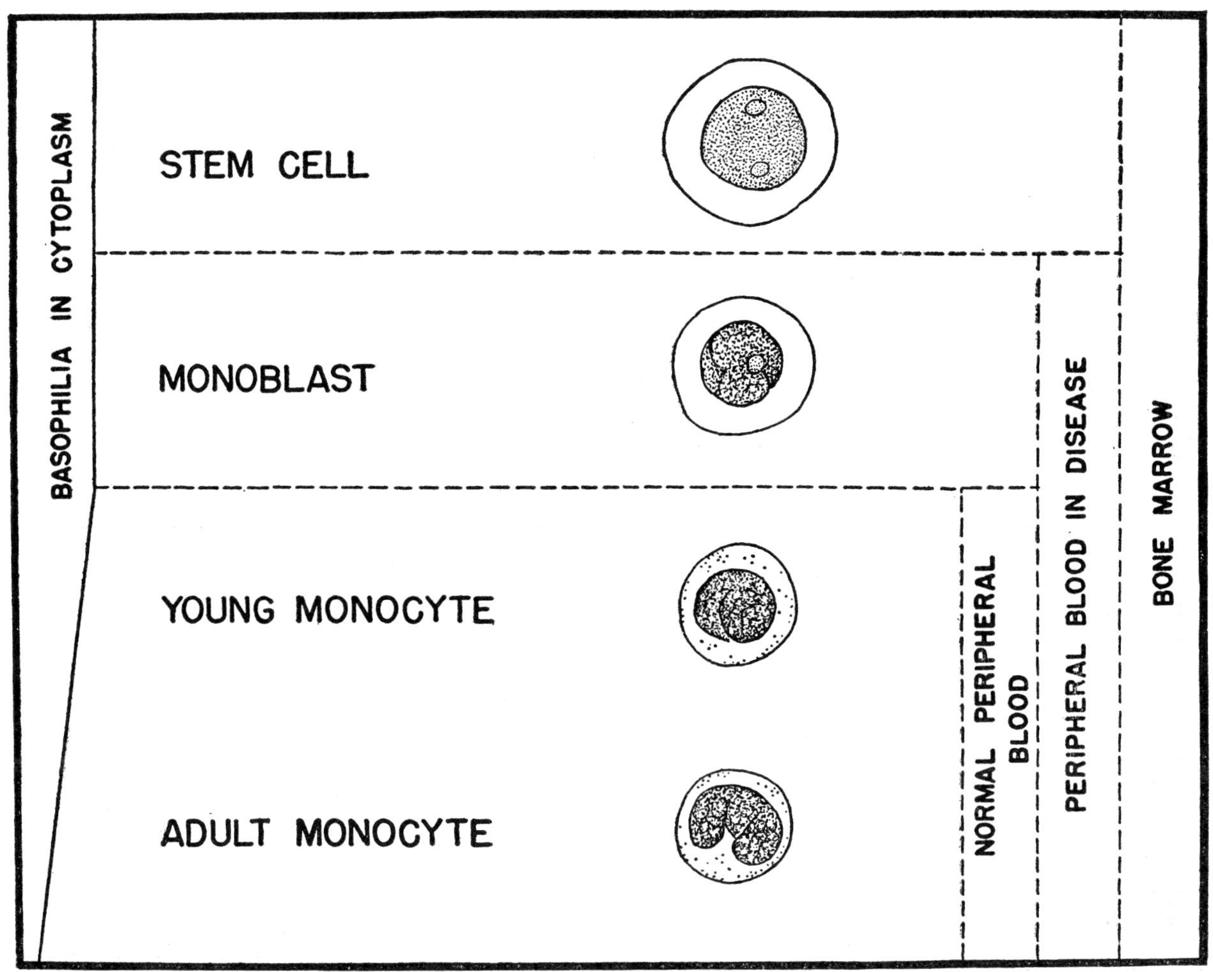

Fig. 7. Diagram of the maturation of the monocytic series.

ender veils. In the cytoplasm there may be vacuoles, as well as phagocytosed red cells, neutrophils, platelets, or cellular debris.

(*c*) Histiocyte — Basophilic or Leukemic Form (Plate XIII). The basophilic form of the histiocyte varies in size, but is larger than the other blasts. The nucleus is often irregular in shape with uniformly granular structure, the granulation being less marked than in the other types of blasts. Nucleoli may or may not be present. The cytoplasm in some cells is deep blue and very irregular in contour; sometimes it is much lighter than would be expected in a cell with a blast type of nucleus. Red-purple granules are often present even in these young forms.

(*d*) Histiocytes — Lymphocytic Form (Fig. 8 and Plate XVI, 4). Large irregular cells with deep-blue cytoplasm often appear in association with an increase of lymphocytes and plasma cells and are usually classified as atypical lymphocytes. It is difficult to identify the origin of these cells in some instances of virus infections, and it is quite probable that they are histiocytes from lymphatic tissue rather than lymphocytes.

(*e*) Histiocytes in Lipoid-Storage Diseases. Large cells, irregular in shape and characterized by the spongy vacuolated cytoplasm, sometimes seen in the lipoid diseases, are histiocytes.

(*f*) "Hemohistioblasts of Ferrata." Ferrata and Franco [93] described a large irregular cell, frequently seen in the blood of patients with chronic myelogenous leukemia, as a hemohistioblast. The light-blue cytoplasm may be clear, spongy, or granular. The type of granules may be eosinophilic, neutrophilic, basophilic, or azurophilic. The nuclear structure is spongelike in character or like a honeycomb. At least one nucleolus is usually present. These are also considered to be tissue cells or histiocytes [245].

7. *DIFFERENTIAL COUNT OF WHITE CELLS.* The differential count of white cells is one of the basic examinations of the patient. It is used for diagnosis and in following the course of the patient. The white-cell count and differential white-cell count in normal individuals, from various sites, are shown in Table 4. The quantitative limitations and significance of the results are discussed by Ham [116], Barnett [13], and others [106, 182, 274]. Normal variations in white-cell counts under basic conditions are given by Stetson [277]. A careful enumeration is made of the white cells on the film, each type of white cell being classified. In order that each cell may be counted only once, the slide is moved progressively and systematically from one field to the next, as much of the film as possible being covered to obtain representative distribution. The number of each class of white cells is determined and the results are expressed in percentage of the total number of white cells enumerated. All abnormal white cells should be classified or described in detail and reported. Some of the different types of abnormal white cells that may be seen in films of peripheral blood have been de-

Fig. 8. Diagram of histiocytes observed in peripheral blood in selected clinical cases.

1. *Subacute bacterial endocarditis.* These histiocytes show evidence of amoeboid activity and phagocytosis. The cell in the center contains a red cell that has been phagocytosed. A red cell is shown in the upper corner for comparative size.

2. *Typhoid fever.* Vacuoles are present in the nuclei.

3. *Reticulum-cell sarcoma.* The histiocytes show vacuolation and evidence of phagocytosis. Nucleoli are present in the two lower cells. A vacuole is present in the nucleus and seven vacuoles occur in the cytoplasm of one of the upper cells. There is vacuole in the cytoplasm of one of the other cells.

4. *Severe anemia.* The histiocytes in this blood film were very irregular in shape, with pseudopods. It can be seen in the upper cell how easily a portion of the cytoplasm can be separated and appear free in the peripheral blood. These cells also show vacuolization.

5. *Hodgkin's sarcoma.* The predominating white cells in this blood film were large cells with deep-blue cytoplasm, containing many vacuoles in both the nucleus and the cytoplasm.

6. *Histiocytic leukemia.* The histiocytes were varied in type in this blood, many showing evidence of amoeboid activity and phagocytosis.

7. *Histiocytic leukemia.* The histiocytes in this case showed evidence of marked amoeboid activity and phagocytosis of red cells (as seen in the cell at the left) and other foreign material (as seen in the two upper cells).

8. *Histiocytic leukemia.* In this blood film, the cells were much larger than a lymphocyte or lymphoblast. The nuclear structure was quite homogeneous but nucleoli were not present. The cytoplasm was deep blue. Evidence of active phagocytosis was seen.

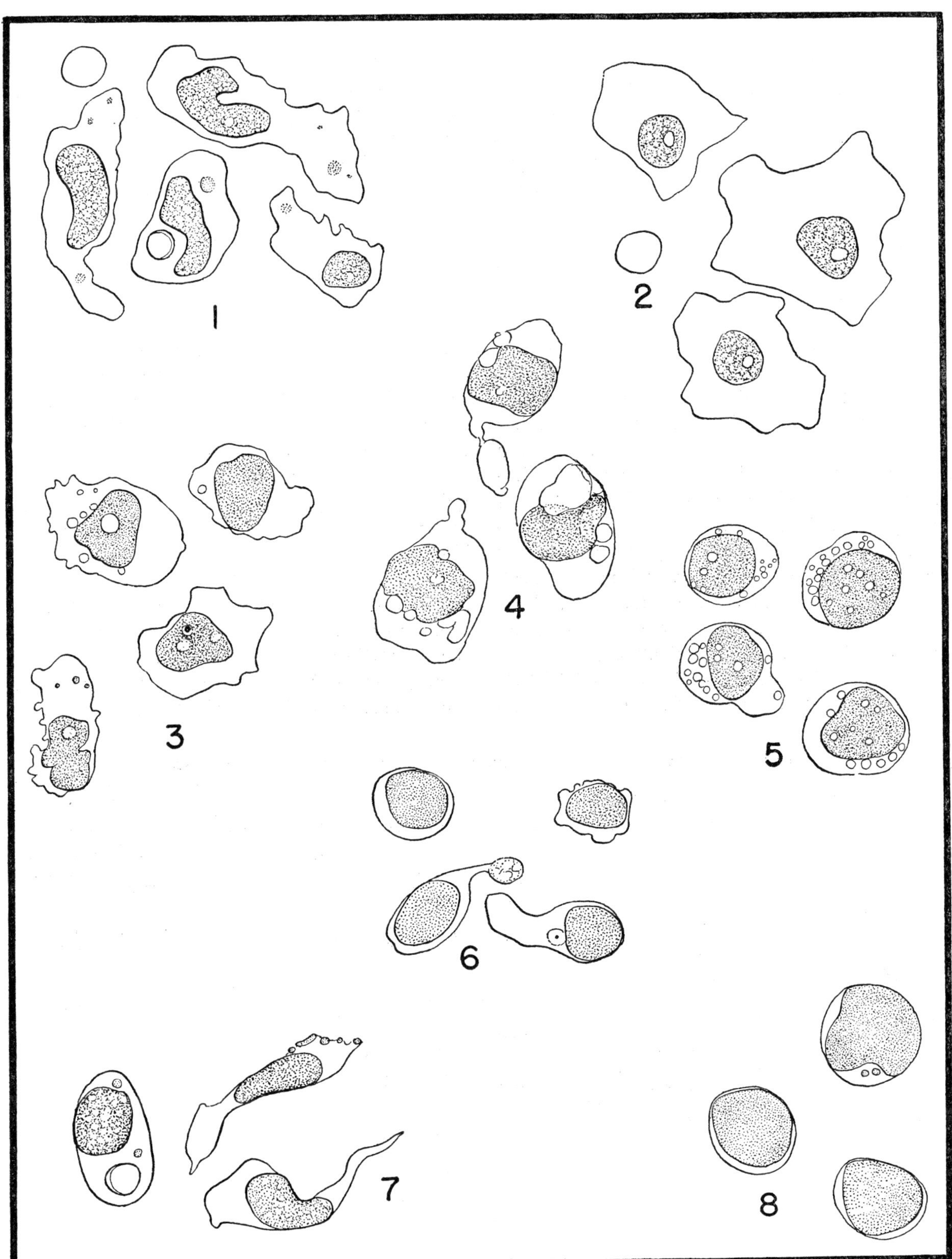

FIG. 8. Diagram of histiocytes observed in peripheral blood in selected clinical cases.

scribed in the preceding paragraphs and are summarized in Table 2. Some other differential points in identifying the early cells are given in the next section. Cells that are ruptured, fragmented, or degenerated ("basket" cells or "smudges") usually cannot be identified and are not included in the differential count, but may be noted separately and reported as the number seen per 100 white cells. A significant number of broken cells may be seen in leukemic bloods. The counts are performed in multiples of 100 cells, using one or two coverglass preparations. At least 100 cells should be counted as a screening procedure.

When nucleated red cells are present in the blood film, they should be reported as the number seen while counting 100 white cells, but they are ***not*** included in the differential count of leukocytes. If there are large numbers of nucleated red cells present, the stage in the erythrocytic maturation series should be noted, an actual count made of the number of nucleated forms per 1000 red cells, and the percentage determined. From this figure the absolute number of nucleated red cells per cubic millimeter is calculated.

8. *DISTINGUISHING CHARACTERISTICS OF IMMATURE CELLS FREQUENTLY CONFUSED.* The recognition of the blast form and its differentiation from the more mature cells is of utmost diagnostic importance. Blasts have in common the characteristics of deeply basophilic cytoplasm, nuclei having finely and homogeneously granular chromatin structure, and frequent presence of nucleoli. In general, the presence of blasts in the peripheral blood is a sign of marked abnormality of the blood-forming organs and should lead to more extensive and repeated blood examinations. Nucleated red cells occurring in the peripheral blood at approximately a normal level of red cells may indicate extramedullary myelopoiesis or myelophthisis due to leukemia, lymphoma, or neoplastic invasion of the bone marrow.

The blasts of red cells should be readily distinguished from the blasts of white cells which often occur in the same blood film, since proerythroblasts or early erythroblasts with basophilic cytoplasm are usually present in association with the more mature nucleated red cells with polychromatophilic or hemoglobin-containing cytoplasm. In the proerythroblast the cytoplasm is more of a deep gray-blue than that seen in the white cells; the nucleus is usually definitely round and more

TABLE 2. CHARACTERISTICS OF CELLS THAT ARE FREQUENTLY CONFUSED

Cells to be distinguished	Diameter (μ)	Cytoplasm		Nucleus				Granules	
		Color	Amount	Shape	Structure	Color	Nucleolus	Color	Number
Monocyte	13–20	Gray-blue	Abundant	*Adult,* Indented *Young,* Round	Reticular, lacy, folded	Blue-purple	0	Purple and red-purple	Few to many, "peppered"
Lymphocyte									
small	7–10	Clear light blue	Scant	Round	Condensed chromatin	Deep purple	0	Red-purple rarely blue	Few, scattered
large	10–20		Abundant	Round		Deep purple	0		
Neutrophil									
adult	10–15	Pink to lilac	Moderate	Segmented	Condensed chromatin	Purple	0	Fine purple	Few to many
young (band)	10–18		Moderate	Not segmented		Purple	0	Fine purple	Few to many
Metamyelocyte	12–20	Pink to lilac	Moderate	Round or indented	Slightly clumped	Purple	0	Fine purple	Few to many
Myelocyte C	15–20	Gray-blue	Moderate	Round	Homogeneous	Purple	0	Purple	Few to many
Histiocyte	15–50	Light gray-blue, spongy	Abundant or irregular	Irregular or round	Honeycomb, vacuolated	Purple	±	Varied, also phagocytic particles	Rare
Plasma cell	10–25	Gray-green-blue	Abundant	Round	Wedges of chromatin	Deep purple	0	0	Rare
Proerythroblast	15–25	Deep blue	Small	Round	Homogeneously granular	Red-purple	+	0	0
Early erythroblast	10–20	Gray-blue	Moderate	Round	Finely divided chromatin	Purple	0	0	0
Late erythroblast	10–20	Blue to lavender	Moderate	Round	Coarse clumping of chromatin	Purple	0	0	0
Normoblast	7–15	Pink to lavender	Variable	Round	Condensed chromatin	Deep purple	0	0	(stippling)

red-purple than in the other blasts; nucleoli may or may not be present.

The recognition of the type of blast of the white-cell series is usually of only academic interest. Identification may be difficult or impossible, and usually contributes little to the welfare of the patient. If blasts are present in association with more mature forms, this is presumptive, but not definite, evidence that the immature cells belong to this same series. Immature cells of the lymphocytic and plasmacytic series may be present in the same blood film in such a disease as infectious mononucleosis. In stem-cell leukemia or in some acute leukemias, because of the abortive cells present, differentiation is not possible. With a leukopenia the number of blast cells may be so small that the identification of the series to which they belong may be impossible. When a " buffy coat " or a concentration of these cells is made before preparing a film, the cells may be distorted so that the series to which the blast belongs cannot be determined. The myeloblast and lymphoblast are quite similar, although the lymphoblast often has less abundant cytoplasm. The plasmablast has the green-blue basophilic cytoplasm that is characteristic of the mature forms of the series. The monoblast is usually larger than either the lymphoblast or the myeloblast; the nuclear structure is more reticular than in the other types of blasts; the nucleus is often folded or irregular in shape; granules are sometimes present in the deep-gray-blue cytoplasm. The size of the cells, the basophilia of the cytoplasm, the structure of the nucleus, and the presence of nucleoli should differentiate the blast forms from lymphocytes which, when mature, have a nucleus about the size of a red cell. For the distinguishing characteristics of other cells that are easily confused, see Table 2.

7. THE PLATELETS AND THE THROMBOCYTIC SERIES

1. *ORIGIN*. Although there have been many theories about the origin of platelets, that presented by Wright [311] has been the most generally accepted. Wright showed that small hyaline bodies containing red-purple granules were detached fragments or pseudopods of the megakaryocytes of the bone marrow that appeared as free formed elements in the peripheral blood. The differential-staining property of Wright's modification [312] of the Romanowsky stain was an important factor in establishing the relation between the granule-containing cytoplasm of the megakaryocyte and the platelets. Other evidence given in support of Wright's theory of platelet formation is: (*a*) platelets are not seen in the embryo until after the appearance of the megakaryocytes; (*b*) blood platelets and megakaryocytes are found only in mammals; (*c*) the number of platelets in the blood roughly parallels the number of megakaryocytes in the bone marrow in certain diseases of physiologic conditions. Wislocki, Bunting, and Dempsey [310] have shown with histochemical methods that there are points of similarity between blood platelets and the cytoplasm of megakaryocytes. The evidence indicates that platelets are cytoplasmic rather than nuclear in origin and probably arise from megakaryocytes.

2. *DESCRIPTION OF NORMAL AND ABNORMAL FORMS OF THE THROMBOCYTIC SERIES* (Fig. 9).

(*a*) Platelet or Thrombocyte. The platelets are formed elements of the blood, measuring 2 to 5 μ in diameter, that appear as a clump of red-purple (azurophilic) granules in a light-blue cytoplasm that is almost transparent. Although true nuclei do not occur in platelets, the granules may be aggregated in a sharply outlined mass in the central part of the platelet, resembling a nucleus. When the blood film is vitally stained with brilliant cresyl blue before the Wright's stain, as for reticulocytes, the cytoplasm is intensely stained with the blue. Sometimes the platelet is devoid of granules, appearing as an irregular mass of cytoplasm. At other times the platelet contains large numbers of granules. The cytoplasm may be intensely blue in some instances, probably a sign of immaturity. These apparently young forms

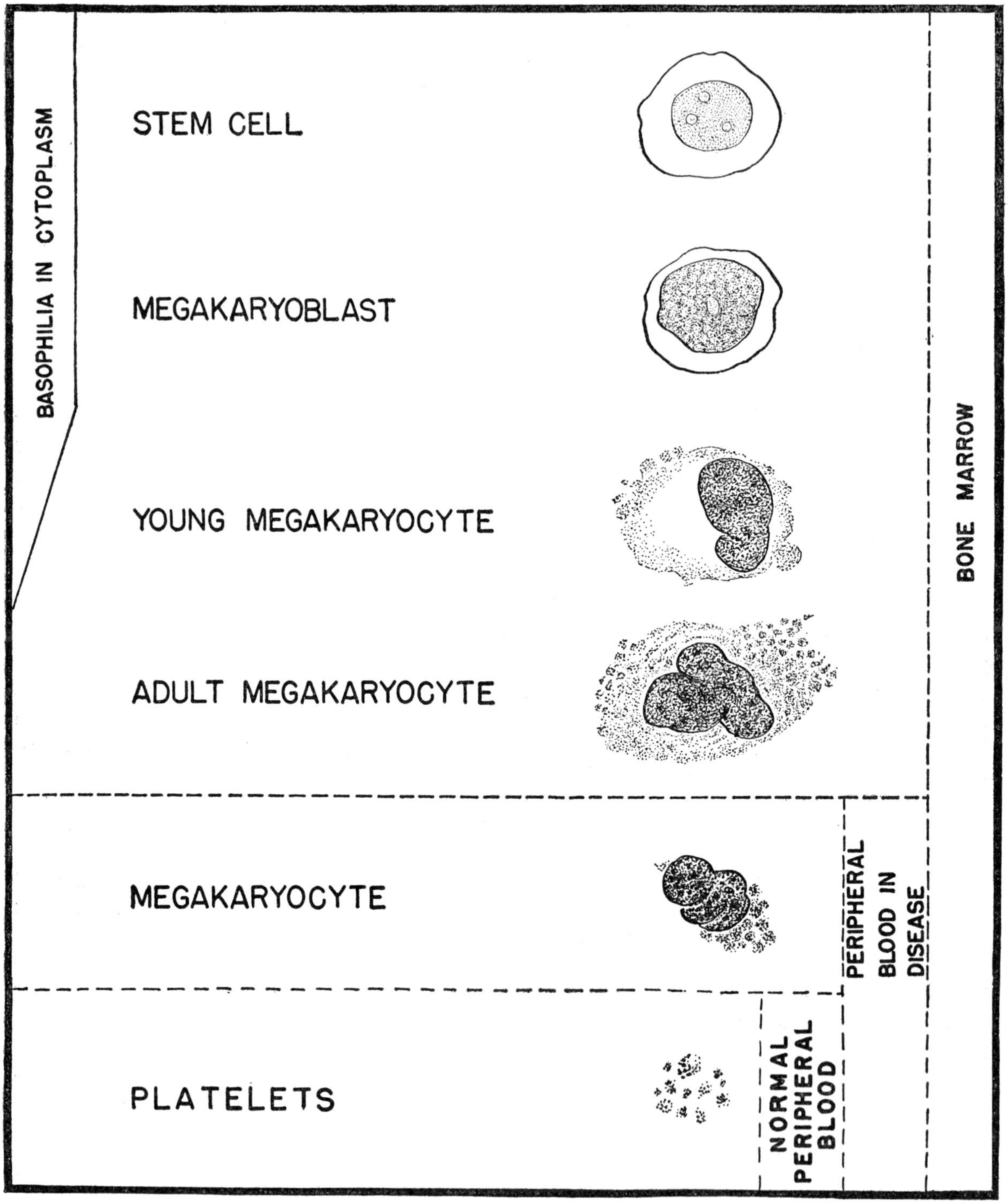

BASOPHILIA IN CYTOPLASM

STEM CELL

MEGAKARYOBLAST

YOUNG MEGAKARYOCYTE

ADULT MEGAKARYOCYTE

MEGAKARYOCYTE

PLATELETS

NORMAL PERIPHERAL BLOOD

PERIPHERAL BLOOD IN DISEASE

BONE MARROW

Fig. 9. Diagram of the maturation of the thrombocytic series. Platelets are shown diagrammatically at the periphery of the megakaryocyte nucleus. (Only platelets are seen normally in the peripheral blood.)

are associated with states of thrombocytopenia or with the sudden increase in number of platelets following hemorrhage or splenectomy [180].

The size of the platelet varies from the normal to abnormally large forms almost the size of a red cell. In normal individuals, approximately 82 percent of the platelets are 2.5 μ in diameter or less [217]. In cases of thrombocytosis, the deviation from normal is usually due to an increase of small platelets. Increase of large platelets is often associated with intense regenerative activity, abnormal function, or hyperplasia of the megakaryocytes in the bone marrow. Although the total number of platelets is abnormally decreased, large platelets are characteristic of the blood picture in aplastic anemia, untreated pernicious anemia, paroxysmal nocturnal hemoglobinuria, chronic lymphocytic leukemia, acute leukemias, or the acute exacerbation of chronic leukemia [167, 291]. Giant platelets are seen in increased numbers in polycythemia vera [194] and in chronic nonleukemic myelosis [37]. Some most unusual forms of platelets have been seen in a few patients with myeloid metaplasia in whom splenectomy had been performed [57].

A decrease in the number of platelets is seen as a result of large doses of benzol, following certain drugs and toxins [83], and following radiation [180]. In infections there may be a decrease of platelets followed by a rapid increase [240, 291]. It is well known that platelets increase rapidly following hemorrhage [217], splenectomy [161, 168] or other surgical operations, childbirth, and fractures [71, 217]. The number of platelets has been increased to more than $1000 \times 10^3/\text{mm}^3$ (normal value, 200 to $400 \times 10^3/\text{mm}^3$) following splenectomy for purpura hemorrhagica [105] and after other surgical procedures. Occasionally an increase in platelets has been associated with postoperative thrombosis and pulmonary embolism [71, 167]. In myelogenous leukemia, the platelets are frequently normal or increased. In 7 of 35 cases in one study [195] the platelets were abnormally increased (800 to $2000 \times 10^3/\text{mm}^3$). When the platelets are increased there may also be many young and abnormal forms of platelets with fragments of megakaryocytes appearing in the peripheral blood. Marked increase or marked decrease from the usual level of platelets in a patient with myelogenous leukemia is a sign of change in the course of the disease.

(*b*) Megakaryocyte (peripheral blood). The megakaryocyte may be seen in the peripheral blood in certain pathologic conditions such as myelogenous leukemia, agnogenic myeloid metaplasia, polycythemia, pneumonia, and sepsis [193]. The nucleus is practically all that is seen of this large distorted cell when it reaches the blood stream. The diameter of the nucleus may vary from that of a red cell to two or three times that of a monocyte. The nucleus of the megakaryocyte has a blue-purple, wavy chromatin structure, with a dark periphery. Sometimes there is a folded or lobulated appearance to the nucleus. The light-blue cytoplasm is rarely seen intact, but appears torn and fragmented, usually containing a mass of blue-purple or azurophilic granules. Platelets that appear as fragments of this granule-containing cytoplasm are often seen in masses attached to or in the vicinity of the megakaryocyte.

(*c*) Megakaryocyte (bone marrow). As indicated by its name, the megakaryocyte is the largest cell of the bone-marrow series (2 to 40 μ), but varies widely in size and appearance. The nucleus is lobulated and is much more dense and deeper blue-purple than the younger cells of the megakaryocyte series. The cytoplasm varies in color from blue to pink and contains a variable number of characteristic red-purple granules. Fragments of cytoplasm are seen breaking off from the cell. Some of these fragments of cytoplasm contain granules and look like platelet material. Platelets are usually associated with these cells.

(*d*) Promegakaryocyte (bone marrow). The promegakaryocyte is smaller than the megakaryocyte. The nucleus is round or beginning to be lobulated. The cytoplasm is more basophilic than in the older form. Granules are present, but are usually fine and scattered around the nucleus.

(*e*) Megakaryoblast (bone marrow). The megakaryoblast is larger than the other blast forms in the bone marrow, but smaller than the adult megakaryocyte. The nucleus is slightly irregular and the chromatin is granular but coarser in structure than in the myeloblast. One or more nucleoli are present. The cytoplasm is relatively small in amount and is deeply basophilic.

(*f*) Abnormal Megakaryocytes (bone marrow). Megakaryocytes with multiple nuclei (polykaryocytes) have been shown to be increased in the bone marrow in pernicious anemia before therapy [89]. These multinucleated megakaryocytes present many abnormal stages of development. There may be hypersegmentation of the nucleus in a cell with basophilic cytoplasm or with mature (pink) cytoplasm. In some thrombocytopenias there is a disturbance of the normal maturation of the megakaryocyte with a preponderance of immature forms, while in other types there is a disturbance of function. For further information the reader is referred to articles on bone-marrow aspirations [54, 69, 101, 170, 237].

3. *EXAMINATION OF PLATELETS IN THE BLOOD FILM.*

(*a*) Method of Determining the Number of Platelets. Counting of platelets by a direct method is preferred whenever it is possible [30, 116, 232]. However the number of platelets can be estimated indirectly by examination of the film of blood stained with Wright's stain to determine semiquantitatively whether the number is increased, normal, or decreased. In this procedure the number of platelets is compared to the number of red cells in the film and will be influenced by the red-cell count. For example, if the red-cell count is $5.0 \times 10^6/\text{mm}^3$ and the platelet distribution on the film appears "normal," this may correspond to an absolute platelet count of $250 \times 10^3/\text{mm}^3$. The same appearance of a "normal" number of platelets relative to the number of red cells on the film may occur in a severe anemia. Thus, if the red-cell count is $1.0 \times 10^6/\text{mm}^3$, an apparently "normal" number of platelets may correspond to an absolute platelet count of $50 \times 10^3/\text{mm}^3$. This is a significant degree of thrombocytopenia which may be observed in pernicious anemia.

(*b*) Clinical Significance. The value of observing the number of platelets in a blood film lies in the detection of an abnormal increase or decrease. The absence of platelets in what appears to be a normal film may confirm a diagnosis of thrombocytopenic purpura when hemorrhagic symptoms are present. The decreased number of platelets in the blood film in the presence of marked red-cell changes may help in classifying the anemia.

8. CASE STUDIES OF VARIOUS DISORDERS OF THE BLOOD

In the following sections, the plates and data are representative of findings from patients in whom the laboratory data are of definite diagnostic value. In these sections the morphologic aspects and clinical interpretations are emphasized. The mechanisms related to the development of anemia are described elsewhere [109, 110, 119, 120, 223]. For a more complete discussion and clinical description the reader is referred to *Clinical Hematology* by Wintrobe [306], *Disorders of the Blood* by W. B. Castle which appears as Chapter 28 in Pathologic Physiology, edited by W. A. Sodeman [39] and *The Haemolytic Anemias, Congenital and Acquired* by Dacie [55].

The following classification, which has been modified from that given by Ham and his associates [117], serves as a guide for the study of the anemias. The illustrative plates are indicated in the outline.

A CLASSIFICATION OF THE ANEMIAS

ANEMIA DUE TO INCREASED LOSS OR DESTRUCTION OF RED CELLS

I. Acute blood loss
   A. Hemorrhage, external (Plate IX)
   B. Hemorrhage, internal (especially into peritoneal cavity)
II. Hemolytic anemia — Increased red-cell destruction
   A. Intracorpuscular abnormalities
      1. Hereditary defects
         (*a*) Hereditary spherocytosis (Plate VII)
         (*b*) Ovalocytosis (homozygous)
         (*c*) Cooley's anemia (Plate V)
         (*d*) Hemoglobinopathies
            (i) Sickle-cell anemia (Plate VI)
            (ii) Hemoglobin C disease
            (iii) Other abnormal hemoglobins

(*e*) Combined defects of hemoglobins or red-cell defects with abnormal hemoglobins (see Table 3)
2. Acquired defect of red cells
(*a*) Paroxysmal nocturnal hemoglobinuria
(*b*) Thermal injury
B. Extra-corpuscular abnormalities
1. Antibodies demonstrable
(*a*) Natural occurring antibodies
Anti-A and anti-B (hemolytic transfusion reaction)
(*b*) Acquired immunity
Rh factor and related blood groups
Favism (no antibody demonstrated)
Drugs: fuadin, quinine
Paroxysmal cold hemoglobinuria
(*c*) "Autoimmunity"
Secondary to leukemia, lymphoma, etc.
Idiopathic
2. Non-immune mechanisms
(*a*) Infectious agents
(i) Red-cell parasitism
Malaria
Oroya fever
(ii) Bacterial toxins or hemolysins
B. Welchii
Hemolytic streptococcus
(*b*) Chemicals
(i) Toxic to normal cells
Arsine
Heavy metals such as lead (Plate IX)
Naphthalein
Phenylhydrazine
Oxidant compounds
Surface acting compounds
(ii) Toxic to susceptible cells — oxidant compounds
Sulfonamides
Primaquine
Phenacetin
(*c*) Congestive splenomegaly
Cirrhosis
Splenic vein thrombosis
(*d*) Unknown mechanisms
Chronic infections
Chronic renal disease
Malignancy

ANEMIA DUE TO DECREASED RED CELL PRODUCTION

I. Nutritional deficiency
A. Deficiency of vitamin B_{12} (macrocytic anemia with megaloblastic marrow)
1. Defective diet
2. Deficiency of gastric intrinsic factor
Pernicious anemia
Total gastrectomy
3. Defective absorption
Sprue
Regional enteritis
Intestinal resection
Tapeworm infestation
B. Deficiency of folic acid (macrocytic anemia with megaloblastic bone marrow)
1. Defective diet
2. Defective absorption
Sprue
Regional ileitis
Intestinal resections
3. Defective utilization
Scurvy
? Cirrhosis
4. Anemia of unknown mechanisms responding to either folic acid or vitamin B_{12} (megaloblastic bone marrow)
"Pernicious anemia" of pregnancy
Megaloblastic anemia secondary to anticonvulsive drugs
Intestinal blind loops
C. Iron deficiency (hypochromic anemia)
1. Increased loss of iron
Chronic hemorrhage
2. Increased requirements for iron
Pregnancy
Growth
3. Decreased intake
Defective diet
Gastric anacidity
Intestinal malabsorption
D. Pyridoxine deficiency
E. ? Protein deficiency
Kwashiorkor

II. Endocrine deficiency
  A. Deficiency of thyroid, adrenal and pituitary hormones
III. Mechanical interference of marrow function
  A. ? Inadequate marrow capacity
    Anemia of newborn
    Anemia of prematurity
  B. Myelophthisis (Plates XI, XII, XIII, XIV and XV)
    Leukemia
    Lymphoma
    Myelofibrosis
    Osteosclerosis
    Metastatic carcinoma
    Primary xanthomatosis
    Miliary tuberculosis
IV. Relative inhibition of marrow
    Chronic infection
    Chronic renal disease
    Cancer
    Cirrhosis
    Collagen diseases
V. Complete bone marrow failure (aplastic or hypoplastic)
  A. Congenital
  B. Acquired
    1. Due to chemicals toxic to normal marrow
      Mitotic poisons (mustards, benzol, etc.)
      Antimetabolites
    2. Due to chemicals toxic to hypersensitive marrow
      Arsenobenzols
      Chloramphenicol
      Gold
    3. Due to physical injury
      Radiation
    4. Idiopathic

9. PLATE III. PERNICIOUS ANEMIA

1. *DESCRIPTION OF UPPER PICTURE: BEFORE TREATMENT (WRIGHT'S STAIN)*. This is definitely the picture of a macrocytic anemia because the average diameter of the red cells is greater than normal (compare with normal cells (*3*) and see also Fig. 1 and Plates I and II). As inspection shows, the variation in size is extreme, from the tiny microcytes (*11*) to oval macrocytes (*9*); the variation in size may be measured according to the method of Price-Jones [234] as shown in Table 1 and Fig. 3. There is marked variation in shape, with many irregular forms (*13*), the most characteristic type being the pear-shaped or tailed forms (*12*). Most of the cells are well filled with hemoglobin, as judged by the depth of staining. A few of the small cells are definitely hypochromic (pale-staining). Polychromatophilic cells (*8*) and stippled cells (*7*) are present. Note that the stippled cells are stained by using Wright's stain alone and are not to be confused with reticulocytes (see lower picture).

There are two white cells in the field — a typical small lymphocyte (*2*) and an abnormally large multilobed neutrophil (*1a*). The platelets (*14*) occur singly and are definitely decreased in number.

2. *DESCRIPTION OF LOWER PICTURE: SIX DAYS AFTER INITIAL TREATMENT WITH LIVER EXTRACT*. The film is stained with brilliant cresyl blue to show the reticulocytes and counterstained with Wright's stain. In this picture the red cells show the same degree of macrocytosis and variation in size and shape as in the upper picture, before treatment. The hemoglobin concentration of the red cells in the lower picture is more variable than in the upper picture, as is evidenced by the variable intensity of staining. This is especially noticeable in the macrocytic reticulocytes, which are sometimes less densely stained than many of the nonreticulated red cells. The red cells containing a network of blue-staining reticulum (*6a, 6b, 6c*) are the reticulocytes. The reticulocytes are numerous, and their age (in the peripheral blood) can be estimated roughly by the amount of reticulum contained in the cells. Thus, a large amount of reticulum (*6a*) indicates the very young cell. As the cell matures, the amount of reticulum decreases (*6b*) until there are only traces of it re-

maining (*6c*). The normoblast (*4*) and erythroblast (*5*) are immature nucleated forms of the erythrocytic series that contain reticulum and should be counted both as reticulocytes and as nucleated red cells (see Plate I).

The white cells in the lower drawing include a normal lymphocyte (*2*) and a normal neutrophil (*1*). The platelets are plentiful.

3. *INTERPRETATION OF BOTH PICTURES.* The marked macrocytosis and extreme variation in size of the red cells are consistent with the diagnosis of pernicious anemia in relapse, in which the variation in size is greater than in any other macrocytic anemia [61]. Among the macrocytes can be seen many oval macrocytes (*9*) that are well filled with hemoglobin. These are especially characteristic of pernicious anemia and are present in large numbers when the red-cell count is very low.

Well-formed microcytes (*11*), full of hemoglobin, and tailed or pear-shaped forms (*12*) are also characteristic of this disease. The number of polychromatophilic red cells (reticulocytes) and nucleated red cells in untreated cases is small, but is increased within about 2 days and reaches the maximum within 7 to 10 days following effective therapy (lower picture) or in spontaneous remission, which rarely occurs. Stippled cells are common, as they are in many severe anemias. Cabot rings and Howell-Jolly bodies in the red cells are found frequently (not illustrated in these pictures).

Before therapy the neutrophils are decreased in number and many of them are abnormally large cells with multilobed nuclei, which are referred to as hypersegmented neutrophils or macropolys. Because of the decreased number of neutrophils, lymphocytes appear to be increased, although their absolute number is within normal limits; this is known as relative lymphocytosis. After effective therapy, the neutrophils quickly return to normal in appearance and in number.

Before therapy the platelets are single, large, and decreased in absolute number; they return to normal following treatment.

When the anemia is severe (red-cell count 0.5 to $2.0 \times 10^6/mm^3$, these abnormal red-cell characteristics are striking, and study of the blood film is of great diagnostic value. However, when the anemia is less severe (red-cell count 2.0 to $3.0 \times 10^6/mm^3$), these features are present to a lesser degree, and the diagnosis is more difficult. At higher levels of the red-cell count (above 3.0 $\times 10^6/mm^3$), some of the abnormal features, such as oval macrocytes, microcytes, tailed forms, stippling, large platelets, and mutilobed neutrophils, may be present, but in decreased numbers.

The macrocytosis and the degree of variation in size of red cells are more striking in Addisonian pernicious anemia than in the other macrocytic anemias that respond to liver extracts, folic acid, and vitamin B_{12}, such as the macrocytic anemias of pregnancy and those of nutritional (extrinsic-factor) deficiency [61].

In the hemolytic anemias, there may be marked macrocytosis and considerable (but not extreme) variation in the size of the red cells in such conditions as severe and chronic acquired hemolytic jaundice, acute exacerbations of chronic hemolytic jaundice, and paroxysmal nocturnal hemoglobinuria. In these conditions, however, without any treatment, the blood film shows marked polychromatophilia (with Wright's stain) and reticulocytosis (with brilliant cresyl blue), as shown in Plate VII. The macrocytes are round and many are polychromatophilic. Oval macrocytes are seldom seen in these hemolytic anemias. The platelets and granulocytes are usually normal and not decreased as in pernicious anemia, except in paroxysmal hemoglobinuria of the nocturnal type.

In certain macrocytic anemias that are " refractory " to liver extract and result from decreased production of red cells, there may occasionally be moderate to marked macrocytosis. This may occur in myelophthisic anemia due to leukemia and in the anemias associated with azotemia and chronic liver disease. In these conditions, the variation in size of red cells is moderate and the number of reticulocytes is low compared to that of the hemolytic anemias.

10. PLATE IV. HYPOCHROMIC ANEMIA (Iron-deficiency Anemia)

1. *DESCRIPTION OF UPPER PICTURE: MODERATE HYPOCHROMIC ANEMIA IN A 17-YEAR-OLD GIRL.* This is the picture of a moderate microcytic anemia with many red cells that are slightly smaller in diameter than the normal cells (*4*). There is moderate variation in shape with a few elongated (pencil) forms (*7*) and a few irregular forms. Microcytes (*6*) are present and one polychromatophilic cell (*9*). The hemoglobin concentration of the red cells is slightly below normal. This may best be judged by comparing the intensity of staining with that of a group of normal red cells as seen in Plate I.

The white cells are normal and include a small lymphocyte (*2*) and a neutrophil (*1*). The platelets (*13*) are normal in number.

2. *DESCRIPTION OF LOWER PICTURE: SEVERE HYPOCHROMIC ANEMIA FROM CHRONIC BLOOD LOSS (HEMORRHOIDS) IN A 62-YEAR-OLD MAN.* Many of the red cells in this drawing are microcytic and hypochromic. However, the variation in size here is extreme, from two large target cells (*8*), which are probably thin cells, to small microcytes (*6*). Also, the variation in shape is extreme, as evidenced by the many irregularly shaped cells and some pencil forms. Polychromatophilic cells (*9*), a normoblast (*11*), and a stippled cell (*10*) are present. Most of the red cells are definitely hypochromic, or low in hemoglobin concentration, as indicated by the pallor of the cells. The hemoglobin appears to be concentrated about the periphery of these thin cells, so that the color seems to decrease gradually from the periphery toward the center. These progressive changes are in contrast to the sharply defined, punched-out areas of central pallor that appear to result from artifacts in fixation or staining of the film.

Two normal white cells are shown in this picture, a neutrophil (*1*) and a monocyte (*3*). The platelets are large and abnormal in shape, as often occurs in a severe anemia, especially of a chronic type. They appear to be approximately normal in number, relative to the red cells on the film, but the platelets may be decreased in absolute number, since the red-cell count is low.

3. *INTERPRETATION OF BOTH PICTURES.* The contrast between these two blood films is so extreme that it suggests different disease processes. However, both represent different degrees of chronic hypochromic microcytic anemia due to iron deficiency. In chronic hypochromic anemia, the greater the anemia, or the lower the hemoglobin concentrations, the more abnormal is the appearance of the red cells.

The upper picture is typical of the changes occurring in the many instances of mild hypochromic anemia. Since the morphologic changes are subtle, the condition may be overlooked. The direct comparison of the patient's blood film with that of a normal person will aid materially in detection of moderate changes (*Atlas*, Section 5, 4a). Also, unless the red cells are well separated on the blood film and well stained, the moderate changes may be missed. However, the lower picture represents extreme changes in the red cells, resulting from chronic iron deficiency due to blood loss over many years.

Usually there is little difficulty in making a correct diagnosis of hypochromic anemia in such cases as those shown here, if the appearance of the blood film is correlated with the red-cell indices and the reticulocyte count. Thus, in both of these cases the values for mean corpuscular volume, MCV, indicated microcytosis and those for mean corpuscular hemoglobin concentration, MCHC, indicated hypochromia. The variation in the diameters is extreme in the lower picture. In both of these cases, the reticulocytes are significantly few, indicating decreased production of red cells by the bone marrow. The level of reticulocytes is lower than would occur in hemolytic anemias, including Cooley's anemia.

4. *OCCURRENCE.* Hypochromic red cells are seen in the film wherever iron deficiency follows blood loss as in neoplasms, ulcers and parasitic infestations of the gastro-intestinal tract and in menorrhagia, etc. In the more severe and chronic conditions the red cells become microcytic as well as hypochromic. Hypochromic anemia may occur when the iron requirements for hemoglobin formation exceed the iron intake during periods of

rapid growth, as in the first year of life, during adolescence, and during pregnancy. Although anemias associated with infections are usually normocytic and normochromic, slightly hypochromic, microcytic anemias may occasionally be found in chronic, active infections such as tuberculosis, rheumatic fever, osteomyelitis and chronic arthritis [306].

Hypochromic microcytic red cells are seen in the blood films of patients with polycythemia vera. These changes in the red cells may be due to previous hemorrhages from ulcers, or to iron deficiency produced by repeated therapeutic venesections.

11. PLATE V. COOLEY'S ANEMIA (Thalassemia Major, Mediterranean Anemia)

1. *DESCRIPTION.* In this picture the red cells show extreme variation in size, shape, and hemoglobin content. A few red cells appear to be normal in size (*4*), but the majority are microcytes. The single most striking feature of the erythrocytes is their extreme variation in shape, which exceeds that usually found in severe anemias and includes many bizarre shapes. Because of the marked variation in the hemoglobin content of cells, there is a marked variation in the intensity of staining of these cells. A few cells appear well filled with hemoglobin, but most of them have a decreased amount of hemoglobin which appears to be distributed around the edge of the cell, as evidenced by the concentration of stained material, such as is seen in hypochromic anemia (Plate IV). Many target forms (*8*) [293] are present. Polychromatophilic cells (*9*) and nucleated red cells are increased. A normoblast with a multilobed nucleus (*13*), a late erythroblast (*14*), and an early erythroblast (*15*) are shown. Cells with Cabot rings (*11*), stippling (*10*), and Howell-Jolly bodies (*12*) are present.

Immature leukocytes include a myelocyte (*3*) and a young lymphocyte (*2*). The platelets (*17*) appear to be normal.

2. *INTERPRETATION.*

(*a*) Cooley's Anemia. This blood film is from a 5-year-old child of Italian parentage, who showed increased fatigability, pallor, recurrent attacks of abdominal pain, mongoloid facies, enlargement of the liver and spleen, and acholuric jaundice.

The changes in the red cells in this picture do not differ greatly (except for the presence of polychromatophilic cells — elevated reticulocytes) from those of severe hypochromic anemia, as seen in the lower picture of Plate IV. From the blood films alone these two conditions may not be distinguishable. However, it is important to recognize, from the data in Tables 6 and 7, that the marked changes in red cells occur at a high level of the red-cell count, $3.3 \times 10^6/mm^3$, and at a hemoglobin level of 5.8 gm/100 ml. Conversely, in the severe hypochromic anemia with comparable red-cell changes, the red-cell count is markedly low, $1.2 \times 10^6/mm^3$, and the hemoglobin level is excessively low, 2.0 gm/100 ml. In Cooley's anemia, the absolute number of reticulocytes is consistently elevated above normal, while in severe hypochromic anemia, untreated, the absolute number of reticulocytes is decreased below normal [29, 300].

This blood film might be confused with that of pernicious anemia because of the marked variation in shape of cells. However, it should be reemphasized that the red cells in Cooley's anemia are hypochromic and microcytic, whereas those of pernicious anemia are normochromic and macrocytic.

(*b*) Cooley's Trait. The blood picture in Cooley's trait is similar to that of a mild hypochromic anemia, showing microcytosis, hypochromia, and moderate variation in size and shape. In addition, there are pencil forms, target forms, frequent stippled cells, rare nucleated red cells, and fewer than 4 percent of reticulocytes. The red-cell count varies from 5.0 to $8.0 \times 10^6/mm^3$, and the mean corpuscular volume is definitely below normal. The values for mean corpuscular hemoglobin concentration are higher, for a given cell size, in Cooley's trait than in hypochromic anemia. A comparison of the blood picture of Cooley's anemia with that of Cooley's trait may well be made by studying Plate IV (hypochromic anemia of iron deficiency), assuming that the red-cell counts are about $5 \times 10^6/mm^3$ in both instances. The final diagnosis depends on the lack of response to iron therapy and a careful study of the blood in other members of the family. Clinically, the subjects with Cooley's trait are usually in normal health, and it is only by careful laboratory studies that the presence of the trait is found. A comparison of the clinical and hematologic findings is given in the report by Daland and Strauss [62].

(*c*) Cooley's Anemia and Cooley's Trait. The genetic relation and the clinical differentiation between Cooley's anemia (thalassemia major) and Cooley's trait (thalassemia minor) have been discussed by many investigators [36, 62, 65, 66, 186, 216, 292, 307]. It is probable that Cooley's anemia is the result of the Cooley factor's being present in the homozygous state, inherited from both parents. The disease is characterized by a severe anemia and is usually considered to be a fatal disease during childhood, but a few cases have been recognized in patients who have survived to the third and fourth decade [62, 183].

Cooley's trait appears to be due to the occurrence of the Cooley factor or gene as a heterozygote. Clinically, the carriers of the trait are asymptomatic although the blood values are abnormal.

Individuals with unusual forms of anemia fulfilling some of the criteria for Cooley's anemia have been observed. These abnormalities are the result of combinations of the Cooley factor and an abnormal hemoglobin. Electrophoresis and various chemical methods now permit the identification of certain abnormal hemoglobins which have been designated by letters in the order of their recognition [243, 271, 276]. Individuals have been found who are simultaneously heterozygous for Cooley's trait and for an abnormal hemoglobin such as: Cooley's factor with hemoglobin S [16, 45, 134, 165, 214, 233, 261, 266, 269], hemoglobin C [266, 267, 315], hemoglobin E [43, 174, 282], and hemoglobin G [258]. In general when two different abnormalities are heterozygous, the clinical and hematologic manifestations are more severe than when either defect is present alone, but not as severe as when either of the abnormal factors is homozygous. The hematologic observations of such cases are summarized in Table 3.

Fetal hemoglobin (hemoglobin F), a normal major constituent of embryonic blood, decreases to less than 5 percent during the first few years of life [140]. In certain pathologic states this fetal hemoglobin remains abnormally high. In Cooley's anemia 50 to 90 percent of the hemoglobin may be of the fetal type [41, 44], as determined by the method of alkali denaturation [264].

The original studies of Minnich *et al.* [192] in Thailand and of Lie-Injo [174] in Indonesia showed a high incidence of apparent Cooley's anemia. Further studies with improved methods revealed the presence of hemoglobin E in some of these families [42, 43, 173, 208]. Some of these individuals were heterozygous for hemoglobin E; some, homozygous for hemoglobin E; and in some the Cooley factor and hemoglobin E were both heterozygous. Homozygous E produces an anemia similar to Cooley's anemia.

Other abnormal hemoglobins such as H and A_2 are found in anemias that are similar to Cooley's anemia and Cooley's trait [4, 163, 204, 246]. Further investigation in this field is in progress.

12. PLATE VI. SICKLE–CELL ANEMIA

1. *DESCRIPTION OF UPPER PICTURE* (unmanipulated film of peripheral blood from a 13-year-old Negro girl). The red cells in this film of peripheral blood show more than normal variation in size. Many of the red cells appear to be a little larger than normal [73] and show more than normal variation in shape, with microcytes, polychromatophilic macrocytes (*5*), and target cells (*6*). The number of crescent or elliptic forms (*7*) and oat-shaped forms is striking; these cells probably represent irreversible sickled forms [259] that have lost their filamentous processes. There is marked variation in hemoglobin concentration, as manifested by the variation in intensity of

TABLE 3. A SUMMARY OF MORPHOLOGIC HEMATOLOGY IN THE HEMOGLOBINOPATHIES

Conditions	Type of hemoglobin [a]	Anemia	Hemoglobin [c] concentration	Size [d]	Reticulocytes	Nucleated red cells	Target forms	Howell-Jolly bodies	Stippling	Sickled forms [e] Fixed prep.	Sickled forms [e] Wet prep.
Sickle-cell trait	A S	0	Norm	Norm	N	0	+	0	0	0	+++
Sickle-cell anemia	S S F [b]	+++	Norm	Norm or Macro	++	++	++	++	++	+ to +++	+++
Sickle-cell and Cooley's	S A F	+++	Hypo	Micro	++	+++	++	+	++	±	+++
Sickle-cell and Hemoglobin C	S C F	+ to +++	Norm	Micro	+	+	+++	+		±	+++
Sickle-cell and Hemoglobin D	S D F	+++	Norm	Macro	++	+	±			+	+++
Sickle-cell and Hemoglobin G	S G	++	Norm	Norm	+		±			+	+++
Hemoglobin C — heterozygous	A C	0	Norm	Norm	N	0	+ to +++			0	0
Hemoglobin C — homozygous	C C F	++	Norm	Norm or Micro	+	±	+++			0	0
Hemoglobin C — Cooley's	C A	+++	Hypo	Micro	+		++			0	0
Hemoglobin D — heterozygous	A D	0	Norm	Norm	N	0	0			0	0
Hemoglobin E — heterozygous	A E	0	Norm	Norm	N	0	0			0	0
Hemoglobin E — homozygous	E E F	+	Norm	Micro	+	±	++			0	0
Hemoglobin E — Cooley's	E A F	++++	Hypo	Micro	++	+++	++			0	0

[a] Hemoglobins included are: A (Adult), F (Fetal), S (Sickle), and C, D, and E.
[b] F represents a value greater than 2 percent.
[c] Norm = normochromic, Hypo = hypochromic.
[d] Norm = normocytic, Micro = microcytic, Macro = macrocytic.
[e] Fixed preparations stained with Wright's stain, wet preparations made with sodium metabisulfite.

staining. The presence of many target cells, which are large thin cells, gives the appearance of a lowered hemoglobin content, although the mean corpuscular hemoglobin concentration (MCHC) is only slightly reduced. The nucleated red cells, which in this film are normoblasts (*8*) and late erythroblasts (*9*), appear in a crisis in sickle-cell disease or may be present in the blood in patients showing chronic anemia of moderate severity.

Only one white cell, a normal lymphocyte (*2*), is shown. Platelets appear to be normal.

2. *DESCRIPTION OF LOWER PICTURE* (film of reduced, anoxic venous blood from a 22-year-old Negro male). Venous blood was reduced by equilibration with 90 percent of nitrogen and 10 percent of carbon dioxide to remove oxygen from the hemoglobin and produce sickling. The film was then made and allowed to dry in a chamber containing the same gas mixture to maintain the hemoglobin in the anoxic form. When a blood film is dried in room air, the sickled forms are well oxygenated and revert to a normal shape. The sickled forms (*7*), stained with Wright's stain, exhibit the great variety of filamentous processes that are seen in unstained wet preparations of blood in which the hemoglobin is reduced by the use of reducing agents such as sodium metabisulfite, ascorbic acid [58], or sodium dithionite [141], or when the oxygen is removed by equilibration with carbon dioxide, or by incubation in a sealed wet preparation for 10 to 24 hours. It is interesting to note that the normoblasts (*8*) and the polychromatophilic cells are sickled (*5*).

The platelets appear to be normal in this film, and one normal neutrophil (*1*) is seen. Obviously, the only cells that sickle are those containing hemoglobin of the abnormal variety found in patients with sickle-cell trait or anemia [229].

3. *INTERPRETATION OF BOTH PICTURES.* The upper picture is from a blood film from a Negro girl who has maintained a red-cell count of 2.0 to 3.5 $\times$ 10^6/mm^3, a hemoglobin level of 6.2 to 9.4 gm/100 ml, and reticulocytosis during a period of nine years of observation. On many occasions, an acute crisis with increased anemia and muscle pains has been precipitated by slight infections. Otherwise, the patient has maintained fairly normal health.

The lower picture is from a Negro male who has maintained a red-cell count of 4.0 to 5.4 $\times$ 10^6/mm^3, a hemoglobin level of 9.5 to 12.6 gm/100 ml, and reticulocytosis during a period of eight years of observation.

4. *SICKLE-CELL ANEMIA AND SICKLE-CELL TRAIT.* The hereditary nature of the sickling phenomenon was recognized in 1917 by Emmel [88], who observed the occurrence of sickling in a father and son on a sealed coverslip preparation of blood. Since then extensive genetic studies have been made which are reported by Neel and

others [6, 209, 210, 211, 212, 262]. They showed that the relation between sickle-cell anemia and sickle-cell trait was due to the presence of the sickling gene as a heterozygote in the trait and as a homozygote in the anemia.

Sickle-cell anemia is usually evident from the blood values and the presence of sickled forms on the blood film. Nucleated red cells, polychromatophilic cells, and target cells are usually present. When the sickling phenomenon is present as a trait, the clinical state and morphologic hematology may be normal. In such cases under abnormal physiologic or pathologic conditions the sickling phenomenon may lead to clinical disorders [50, 205]. In 1927 [114], Hahn and Gillespie showed that sickling is a reversible phenomenon, depending on the degree of oxygenation of the hemoglobin. In the homozygous state the erythrocytes contain enough of the abnormal hemoglobin (hemoglobin S) to allow sickling within the physiologic range of oxygen tensions, but in heterozygous form the oxygen tension must be abnormally diminished to cause sickling. The sequence of events in the pathologic physiology of this disease state is discussed by Harris and coworkers [120]. Whenever hemoglobin S is present, sickling can be demonstrated by reducing the oxygen tension artificially and thus increasing the percentage of sickled forms and the viscosity [109]. The simplest method for the demonstration of sickling is the use of a reducing agent such as 2-percent sodium metabisulfite [58]. One or two drops of a freshly prepared solution is mixed with one drop of blood on a slide and covered with a coverglass on which pressure is momentarily exerted to extrude excess blood and produce a thin film. This preparation is examined under high-dry power of the microscope immediately and for at least 15 min. As many as 80 to 100 percent of the red cells may show these filamentous sickled forms during this period. Sometimes the sickle cells appear more like a holly leaf in shape. A positive result indicates the existence of a moiety of hemoglobin S whether in the homozygous or heterozygous state. The bisulfite test is the most effective and practical method of effecting deoxygenation and of evoking sickling. It is a useful screening test to determine the incidence of sickling among Negro or other populations and for genetic, epidemiologic, and ethnic studies [169, 213].

5. *HEMOGLOBINOPATHIES.* When Pauling and co-workers [229] introduced the electrophoretic method of studying hemoglobin, a new field was opened up. Not only has a better understanding of the sickle-cell disease been attained, but other abnormal hemoglobins have been observed. To date, in addition to the normal adult hemoglobin (A) and fetal hemoglobin (F), hemoglobin S, C, D, E, G, H, I, J, and K have been observed [41, 140, 262, 302, 316]. Hemoglobin S as a heterozygote has been observed in combination with hemoglobin C [215, 235], hemoglobin D [153, 154, 281], and hemoglobin G [258], as well as with the Cooley trait (p. 36). Hemoglobin F is present in increased amounts in many of these hemoglobinopathies. Some of the morphologic observations are shown in Table 3. Observations on variants of sickle-cell disease are discussed by Griggs and Harris [110].

In the homozygous state hemoglobin C is associated with a mild anemia, the most striking feature morphologically being the presence of target cells [121, 256, 263, 271, 284]. Target cells are evident in the blood film in the C trait but anemia is absent.

Generalizations about the abnormal hemoglobins D, G, H, I, J, and K are not possible because of the limited number of cases observed at the present date.

13. PLATE VII. HEMOLYTIC ANEMIA — CHRONIC AND ACUTE

1. *UPPER PICTURES: CHRONIC HEMOLYTIC JAUNDICE — HEREDITARY SPHEROCYTOSIS* (two films from the same sample of blood; the *left-hand* film is stained with Wright's stain; the *right-hand* film is stained with brilliant cresyl blue and counterstained with Wright's stain).

(*a*) Description. The red cells show moderate variation in size although the average size is about normal. This variation in size results from the presence of three types of cells: normal red cells (*8*), spherocytes (*9*), and large polychromatophilic cells (*10*) in the left-hand and reticulocytes (*11*) in the right-hand pictures. The spherocytes are small, round, and intensely stained, and are characteristic of this disease, which is also called hereditary spherocytosis. The variation in intensity of staining is the striking feature in these two films. The larger cells that are polychromatophilic (*10*) and the reticulocytes (*11*) are slightly less intensely stained than the normal cells (*8*), as is often the case with these newly formed cells. The spheroidal cells are hyperchromic and, because of their shape, lack the central pallor of the normal biconcave red cell.

Normal white cells are present, namely, monocytes (*6*), neutrophils (*1*), and eosinophils (*5*). The platelets appear normal.

(*b*) Clinical Discussion. These blood films were obtained from a patient with typical congenital hemolytic jaundice who refused splenectomy. He has been under observation for 20 years with chronic anemia and reticulocytosis. Except for four episodes of biliary obstruction when jaundice was intense with bilirubinuria, the patient has had moderate icterus and acholuria. His red-cell count has varied from 3.0 to 4.5 $\times$ 10^6/mm^3, and his hemoglobin from 7.8 gm to 10.9 gm/100 ml. The reticulocytes have fluctuated between 5 and 20 percent. The osmotic and mechanical fragilities of the red cells have been increased. Similar findings should also be manifest in at least some members of the patient's family.

2. *LOWER PICTURE: ACUTE HEMOLYTIC ANEMIA—SULFANILAMIDE INTOXICATION* (with leukemoid reaction).

(*a*) Description. The red cells show more variation in size than in the upper drawings. Polychromatophilic macrocytes (*10*), spherocytes (*9*), and normal cells (*8*) are present. In addition, there are irregular forms (*13*) and nucleated red cells—normoblast (*14*) and late erythroblast (*15*). In addition to the appearance of young red cells in this film, there are immature white cells of the granulocyte series — band neutrophil (*2*), metamyelocyte (*3*), and myelocyte (*4*). A normal monocyte (*6*) and a small lymphocyte (*7*) are also present. The platelets are increased in number.

(*b*) Clinical Discussion. The lower picture was obtained from the blood film of a 23-year-old man, who, because of scarlet fever, was treated with sulfanilamide for only 3 days. On the fourth day, the patient had marked hemoglobinemia and hemoglobinuria, with a decrease in red-cell count to 1.3 $\times$ 10^6/mm^3 and in hemoglobin to 4.4 gm/100 ml. There was an increase in the white-cell count to 54 $\times$ 10^3/mm^3, with a myeloid response of the granulocytic series and an increase in immature forms of the erythrocytic series appearing in the peripheral blood. There was an increase of reticulocytes to 8.4 percent, an increased mean corpuscular volume (111 μ^3), and increase in the osmotic fragility of the red cells. The icterus index could not be read because of hemoglobinemia, but the bilirubin was elevated, as shown in Table 9. The number of nucleated red cells increased to 10 per 100 white cells. Howell-Jolly bodies and stippled cells, though not shown in the plate, were present, as well as the polychromatophilic cells.

The patient recovered promptly, after transfusions, from this fulminating episode of hemolytic anemia, which was characterized by intravascular hemolysis, increased osmotic fragility of the red cells, and a marked physiologic response of the bone marrow.

3. *INTERPRETATION.* The blood pictures in these two hemolytic anemias have a great deal in common. In both conditions the peripheral blood shows polychromatophilic cells (or, when vitally stained, reticulocytes), normal cells, and spherocytes. Both cases had an increased osmotic fragility of the red cells consistent with the presence of spherocytes. In one patient, there was abnormal icterus (bilirubinemia); in the other, hemoglobinemia and hemoglobinuria.

The blood picture in the acute hemolytic anemia is more abnormal than in the chronic hemolytic jaundice, as evidenced by the presence of immature granulocytes, nucleated red cells, and the fragmented red cells and half-moon shapes. Such a striking change in blood picture may also be seen in acute hemolytic anemia resulting from a variety of causes such as naphthalene poisoning, thermal burns, hemolytic transfusion reactions, or acquired hemolytic jaundice [55, 118, 260].

14. PLATE VIII. ERYTHROBLASTOSIS FETALIS

1. *DESCRIPTION.* The red cells in this film are definitely macrocytic, with some variation in size but very little variation in shape. The macrocytes, whether mature forms or immature forms, are round (compare with the oval macrocytes in pernicious anemia, Plate III). The cells are well filled with hemoglobin. There are many polychromatophilic cells (*8*), nucleated red cells of all stages (*11–15*), stippled cells (*9*), and Howell-Jolly bodies (*10*). Young cells of the granulocytic series (*2, 4*) are present in addition to the normal neutrophil (*1*) and lymphocyte (*3*). Platelets appear to be about normal in number and size.

2. *INTERPRETATION.* This blood film is from a newborn infant who died of erythroblastosis fetalis 16 hours after birth. The red-cell count was $1.5 \times 10^6/\text{mm}^3$; the hemoglobin, 6.2 gm/100 ml. The spleen and liver were markedly enlarged. The infant's Rh-positive red cells were sensitized by anti-Rh antibody from the mother. In this particular family, there was a classic incidence of erythroblastosis fetalis with death of four infants — all but the first child. This indicates that the paternal blood group was homozygous Rh positive.

This blood picture can be differentiated morphologically from other macrocytic anemias, because there is more variation in size here than in any other of the anemias except possibly pernicious anemia. The picture is *not* characteristic of pernicious anemia, because the macrocytes are not oval, there is comparatively little variation in shape, and there is much more polychromatophilia than is seen in untreated pernicious anemia.

The presence of many polychromatophilic cells and nucleated red cells is consistent with the physiologic response of the bone marrow in subacute or chronic hemolytic anemia. An acute hemolytic anemia does not usually show such a marked macrocytosis (compare Tables 9 and 10). However, the red cells in the newborn infant are normally macrocytic, are well filled with hemoglobin [206], and show moderate polychromatophilia. The mean red-cell diameter in the normal infant is 8.6 μ. The macrocytosis and reticulocytosis or erythroblastosis due to the hemolytic reaction are added, therefore, to the normal macrocytosis of the infant's blood cells. In addition, in an infant or child, because of the large volume of active bone marrow, any extra demand on the marrow readily produces immature cells of the erythrocytic and granulocytic series that appear in the peripheral blood.

15. PLATE IX. ACUTE BLOOD LOSS; CHRONIC LEAD POISONING

1. *UPPER PICTURE: ACUTE BLOOD LOSS* (physiologic response of bone marrow).

(*a*) Description. The red cells show slightly more than normal variation in size. The average size of the new young polychromatophilic cells (*7*) is slightly increased and there are some cells present that are slightly smaller than the normal cells (*4*); there is practically no variation in shape. The hemoglobin content of the cells is about normal. One target cell is present (*9*). The white cells include a typical neutrophil (*1*) and monocyte (*3*). The platelets (*10*) are about normal in number, but some are large.

(*b*) Interpretation. This is the blood picture in a young woman, 25 years of age, ten days after the onset of acute blood loss from menorrhagia. There was no evidence of chronic blood loss. The polychromatophilic cells (reticulocytes 9 percent, Plate IX and Table 11) represent the immature red cells which appeared in the peripheral blood as a normal physiologic response to the acute blood loss in a patient without iron deficiency. At the time when these young red cells are present in increased numbers, the mean corpuscular volume is increased (104 μ^3) and the mean diameter of the cells is also greater than normal.

The variation in size might be confused with that observed in moderate hypochromic, microcytic anemia (Plate IV, upper picture). However, the red-cell indices in this patient show slight macrocytosis and normochromic red cells. Also, the cells of this blood film, when compared with those of a normal blood, are seen to be well filled with hemoglobin. Hemolytic anemia must be considered because of the presence of polychromatophilic cells, the slight macrocytosis, and the variation in size. The normal icterus index is evidence against increased destruction of red cells, but does not exclude it completely. The final diagnosis depends upon the recovery from the anemia with or without administration of iron therapy.

2. *LOWER PICTURE: CHRONIC LEAD POISONING.*

(*a*) Description. The red cells in this blood film appear normocytic with slight variation in size but very little variation in shape. The hemoglobin concentration of the cells is normochromic. The striking abnormality here is the presence of a large number of stippled cells (*8*) and polychromatophilic cells (*7*). Stippling may occur in either the adult red cell or the younger form (polychromatophilic cell). The stippling is observed in a film stained with Wright's stain alone and does not require staining with brilliant cresyl blue. Stippling should not be confused with the reticulum of young red cells (see Plate I), which does require brilliant cresyl blue for its demonstration. The stippling varies in degree from coarse granules to fine punctate material.

The white cells include a normal neutrophil (*1*) and lymphocyte (*2*). The platelets (*10*) appear normal.

(*b*) Interpretation. Although the presence of stippled cells alone does not necessarily indicate chronic lead poisoning, the occurrence of stippled cells and polychromatophilic cells, associated with normal or slightly hypochromic red cells, does suggest lead poisoning. According to the data in Table 11, there is a moderate, normocytic anemia with increased reticulocytes (8 percent) and a normal icterus index. Accordingly, the large number of stippled cells, which represent 2.8 percent of the red cells, serves as a clue to distinguish this case from that of acute blood loss (upper picture) or hemolytic anemia. Stippled cells, however, are also characteristic of Cooley's trait and of many other anemias, but usually are fewer in number and are associated with other changes in the red cells. The diagnosis of chronic lead poisoning may be confirmed by the history of exposure to lead and by demonstrating an abnormal excretion of lead and coproporphyrin in the urine [116, 297]. Since the type of porphyrin excreted in lead poisoning is abnormal, it is possible that the stippling of the red cells is an expression of a disturbance in metabolism or retardation of the formation of hemoglobin [297]. The anemia does not respond to the usual antianemia therapy.

16. PLATE X. LEUKOCYTOSIS

1. *DESCRIPTION OF BOTH PICTURES. UPPER PICTURE:* Leukocytosis, associated with carcinoma of the lung; *LOWER PICTURE:* Leukocytosis with toxic manifestation due to overwhelming sepsis.

In both of these patients the peripheral blood showed a definite leukocytosis, increase in the count being due to the cells of the granulocytic series. The predominating cell is the young neutrophil or band form (*2*). In the pictures there are only two adult neutrophils (*1*) present, the essential requirement for the adult form being two or more lobes of the nucleus connected by a thread. In these pictures younger cells of the granulocytic series are also present: metamyelocyte (*3*), myelocyte C (*4*), and myelocyte B (*5*). These bands and metamyelocytes, which are often larger in infectious conditions than in normal blood, should be compared with the monocytes (*8*) for contrast in staining reactions and structure. The difference between the lacy structure of the nucleus in the monocytes (*8*) and the homogeneous chromatin of the myelocytes is very well shown, as is also the difference in the intensity of the blue of the cytoplasm. The young neutrophils or bands (*2*) and the metamyelocytes (*3*) in the lower picture show large toxic granules and marked vacuolization of the cytoplasm. One of the cells (*2a*) shows a Döhle body. A plasma cell (*10*) and a histiocyte (*9*) are present as well as lymphocytes (*6, 7*). In the case shown in the upper picture the white-cell count was 35,000/mm^3, with 95 percent of the cells in the granulocytic series. In the case shown in the lower picture, the white-cell count was 29,000/mm^3, although in such a toxic condition the white-cell count may be depressed. The red cells appear normochromic in both cases, and they are slightly macrocytic in the lower picture. The platelets appear increased in the upper picture, as is usual with a normal response of the bone marrow; they appear to be decreased in the lower picture, a fact which has a grave prognosis in infection.

2. *INTERPRETATION*. The granulocytic response as shown in the upper picture is typical of a physiologic response to exercise, mild infection especially with pyogenic organisms, acute blood loss, acute hemolytic anemia, convulsions, infarcts, thrombosis, diabetic acidosis, uremia, certain drug intoxications, carcinoma, tissue necrosis, polycythemia vera, and after splenectomy.

The granulocytic response as seen in the lower picture is much more severe and abnormal. This is a picture of overwhelming sepsis and indicates a grave prognosis. There are no adult neutrophils in the picture. An increase in young forms has been termed a " shift to the left " by Arneth [9], Schilling [254], and others, but actually it means a " shift to immaturity " with a reduction of the marrow threshold with liberation of increased numbers of young forms. Many classifications and hemograms have been used to interpret the meaning of the changes in the maturity of the cells. It is essential to differentiate the mature forms of granulocytes (cells in which the nucleus has two or more lobes connected by a thread) from the immature forms with band, indented, or round nucleus (bands, metamyelocytes, and myelocytes). This increase of immature cells may be termed a " regenerative shift " which is the normal physiologic response, or a " degenerative shift " in cases in which there is a depression of the bone marrow with an insufficient supply of the neutrophils in the peripheral blood to meet the needs. The degree of immaturity indicates the severity of the reaction. In severe reactions, when myelocytes and immature red cells appear in the peripheral blood, the term " myeloid response " is used. Leukemoid responses have been reported in septicemia [160], in chronic and acute infections [81, 275], acute hemolytic anemia [124, 129, 287], and in acute blood loss [57]. The presence of heavy blue-black granules in the neutrophils, bands, and metamyelocytes, as seen in the lower picture, is an indication of severe infection or necrosis [108, 162]. These toxic granules are usually present in pyogenic infections, certain viral infections, necrosis, malignant tumors, and liver disease. Marked vacuolization, as seen in some of the cells in the lower picture, is usually considered to be a stage in the disintegration of the cells. This is often seen in the cells in overwhelming infections. This vacuolization should not be confused with that present in the cells when the films are made from blood preserved with an anticoagulant. Döhle bodies were described by Hill [130] in cases of streptococcal infections, but subsequent observations have shown that they may be present in other types of severe infections. The qualitative changes in the white cells are fully as important in interpreting the blood picture as the quantitative changes. Plasma cells (*10*) and histiocytes (*9*) are frequently seen in response to increased demand on the blood-forming tissue.

3. *LEUKOCYTOSIS IN INFANTS AND CHILDREN*. The normal baby at birth may have a leukocytosis of 10.0 to 45.0×10^3/mm^3. This white-cell count decreases during the first 26 weeks. Children may have a white count slightly greater than adults. Osgood and associates [220] in a study of 86 children from 4 to 7 years of age found a mean value for white cells of $10.419 \pm 0.176 \times 10^3$/mm^3, with 95 percent of the observations showing a range of 5.5 to 15.5×10^3/mm^3. The bone marrow in infants and children is more active than in the adult. Therefore, for a given response, the increase in the white count is greater and the presence of immature granulocytes and erythrocytes in the peripheral blood does not imply as serious a prognosis as it would in an adult. A myeloid reaction in an in-

fant with pneumonia was reported by Buckman [33] in which the white-cell count rose to $84.5 \times 10^3/\text{mm}^3$ with 9 percent myelocytes. There were nucleated red cells and megakaryocyte fragments in the peripheral blood.

4. *LEUKOPENIA.* The mechanism of leukopenia may involve decreased production by the bone marrow, redistribution after delivery to the circulation, or increased loss or destruction of the cells. The total white-cell count may be decreased with a decrease of neutrophils either relative or absolute. The neutrophils that are present are usually young forms. In certain conditions the neutrophils may be decreased in absolute number with a relative increase of band forms and perhaps metamyelocytes. Such changes have been seen in bacterial endocarditis, miliary tuberculosis, and paroxysmal nocturnal hemoglobinuria. Neutropenia may be due to depression of the bone marrow as the result of toxic action of or hypersensitivity to certain drugs and chemicals such as benzol, amidopyrine, dinitrophenol, the sulfonamides, thiouracil, and chloramphenicol [46, 155, 164, 171, 295]. Neutropenia may be the result of replacement of the normal marrow with foreign cells as in metastatic carcinoma, xanthomatosis, or fibrous tissue. Neutropenia with a relative lymphocytosis is usually seen in pernicious anemia and in certain other conditions where there is a known nutritional deficiency. Neutropenia is the usual response of the bone marrow to anaphylactic shock. The association of splenomegaly and sometimes hepatomegaly with neutropenia has been considered by Wiseman and Doan [309] as a separate entity called primary splenic neutropenia. Cyclic neutropenia has also been reported [52, 222, 247].

5. *AGRANULOCYTOSIS.* This disorder is characterized by an acute course, fever, necrotic lesions of the mucous membranes, leukopenia, and severe granulocytopenia. In such cases the platelets and red cells are usually normal with the striking changes affecting only the granulocytic series. The association of agranulocytosis with sensitivity to drugs has been demonstrated by many authors [68, 144, 181]. A case of agranulocytosis was reported by Jackson *et al.* [143] in which there was a periodic decrease in the neutrophils associated with the menstrual cycle. More recent work has demonstrated an immunologic agranulocytosis [70, 198].

6. *EOSINOPHILIA.* An increase in white-cell count with an absolute increase of eosinophils occurs in allergic diseases, parasitic infestations, skin diseases, neoplastic disease, periarteritis nodosa, and Loeffler's syndrome, and during the recovery phase in many infections. It is interesting that multilobed eosinophils are often seen in these responses of the bone marrow, while the eosinophil with a bilobed nucleus is usually seen in the normal blood [57, 253].

7. *EOSINOPENIA.* It has been well recognized clinically that an early sign of severe infection, especially by pyogenic organisms, is the disappearance of the eosinophils from the peripheral blood; conversely, a sign of recovery is their reappearance [242, 303]. Eosinopenia is considered a regular manifestation in such conditions as shock, major surgical procedures, and Cushing's disease, and following the injection of certain adrenal cortical hormones [131, 289].

8. *BASOPHILS.* The number of basophils in the peripheral blood is low (0 to 2 percent); therefore, there is no clinical significance to the absence of basophils. However, they usually disappear during severe infection and reappear with recovery as do the eosinophils. Increase of basophils is a frequent finding in myelogenous leukemia, myeloid metaplasia, and polycythemia vera. In leukemia the relative number of basophils may be exceedingly high following radiation, but the absolute number may be the same as the pretreatment level.

9. *HEREDITARY ANOMALIES OF THE WHITE BLOOD CELLS.*

(*a*) Pelger-Huët Familial Anomaly. In this condition, first described by Pelger, the neutrophils of the peripheral blood have bilobed nuclei, while the number of band forms is increased. Metamyelocytes and myelocytes are occasionally seen. The chromatin structure of the nucleus of the neutrophils appears clumped as in a mature cell, while the nuclear form is immature. Individuals with this abnormality are clinically normal and respond to infection and other demands on the bone marrow with an increase of immature granulocytes. Huët, in 1932 [133], produced evidence that this anomaly occurred in families.

Since then the dominant hereditary nature has been confirmed by other investigators [20, 159, 290].

(*b*) Hereditary Granulation Anomaly. Alder [5] first described the occurrence of abnormal coarse blue-black granules in the neutrophils of individuals who had no infection or known disease. This abnormal granulation was present in the neutrophils and eosinophils, as well as in the younger cells of the granulocytic series. This condition was observed by Alder repeatedly in one woman over a period of 8 years and in two members of another family. Jordans [152] has studied a family in which this granulation anomaly was observed in many members of one family, representing three generations.

(*c*) Familial Eosinophilia. Several reports [7, 278] may be found in the literature in which an increase of eosinophils was present in several members of a family. When no other cause for the eosinophilia is found, this is considered a familial anomaly.

17. PLATE XI. MYELOGENOUS LEUKEMIA

1. *DESCRIPTION OF BOTH PICTURES.* The pictures represent blood films from two patients with chronic myelogenous leukemia.

(*a*) White Cells. By a study of these plates, practically all the typical cells in the development of the granulocytic series can be identified. In the upper picture there are two neutrophils (*1*) and two young neutrophils or band forms (*3*). One of these band forms is much younger than the other and by some might be classed as a metamyelocyte. The nucleus, however, has two lobes connected by a band, like a dumbbell. The character of the nucleus is mature, with clumped chromatin. A typical eosinophil (*2*) is shown with large discrete red-orange granules. Three basophilic cells (basophils) are present — a young basophil (*5*), an abnormal form (*6*), and a basophilic myelocyte (*12*). The basophilic granules in the myelocyte B (*12*) should be contrasted with the neutrophilic granules of myelocyte B (*10*). The dark-blue basophilic granules are definitely larger than those of the neutrophilic myelocyte (*10*), but are usually smaller than the basophilic granules in the more mature basophils (*5* and *6*). Eosinophilic myelocytes (*11*) are striking because of the large red-orange granules which cover the round nucleus. The granules in one of the eosinophilic myelocytes do not have their full color, although they are large. (In other patients with myelogenous leukemia, the eosinophilic myelocytes frequently contain granules that are smaller than those shown in Plate XI. Occasionally, both eosinophilic and basophilic granules occur in the same cell.) There is considerable contrast between the eosinophilic myelocyte B (*11*) and the more mature forms — the eosinophilic myelocyte C (*9*), young eosinophil (*4*), and adult eosinophil (*2*).

In the lower picture all stages of the neutrophilic series of granulocytes are shown. The typical myeloblast (*14*) is shown with a fine granular nucleus containing a nucleolus, and surrounded by a rim of deeply basophilic cytoplasm, without granules. A similar cell (*13*) with a typical " blast " nucleus and basophilic cytoplasm, but containing nonspecific, azurophilic granules, is called a myelocyte A, or early myelocyte. By many observers, this could be considered a blast because of the nucleolus. The granules in the cytoplasm are not differentiated into neutrophilic, basophilic, and eosinphilic types until the cell is at a more mature stage (myelocyte B). The myelocyte B of all types has already been described (*10, 11, 12*). The myelocyte C, containing neutrophilic granules (*8*), has the same type of nucleus and cytoplasm as the neutrophilic myelocytes of stage B (*10*). However, the granules, which are scattered throughout the cytoplasm, do not cover the nucleus. The homogeneous nuclear structure and the light gray-blue color of the cytoplasm are the same in both the myelocyte B and the myelocyte C. Occasionally, the granules in the myelocyte C are absent or poorly stained, although this stage of development may be identified by comparing it with the myelocyte B of the same film. The metamyelocyte (*7*) should not be confused with the myelocyte C (*8*), since the cytoplasm of the metamyelocyte has acquired the pink-lavender color of the neutrophil with a nucleus that is beginning to show slight condensation of chromatin. This metamyelocyte may be compared with the band form and adult neutrophil in the same film for the color of the cytoplasm. In the young neutrophil (*3*), the two lobes of the nucleus are distinct but connected by a thick band, whereas in the adult form of the neutrophil the lobes of the nucleus are separated by threads of chromatin.

The young form of the monocytic series (*15*), shown in the upper picture, is often confused with the metamyelocyte (*7*) or the late myelocyte (*8*). However, the young monocyte with a round nucleus has the same lacy or reticular structure of the nucleus and often the same folded or fissured outline of the nuclear chromatin as in the lobulated nucleus of the mature monocyte (see Plate II, *10*). These cells may best be differentiated by comparison with known cells of the same series in the same film. The young monocyte should be compared with the adult monocyte for size, nuclear structure, color of the cytoplasm, and type of granulation. The myelocyte C should be compared with the myelocyte B of the same film. The nuclear structure of these cells, as shown in Plate XI, is quite different. Thus, the monocyte has a reticular, fissured nucleus, the metamyelocyte shows the first stages in the condensation of the chromatin that occurs as the cell matures, whereas the myelocyte C has a homogeneous nucleus. Similarly, the cytoplasm of each of the three varieties of cells should be compared with that of the others and of related cells of the same series. Monocytes and lymphocytes are usually present in the blood film in myelogenous leukemia, but the relative number is small since the increase is due to cells of the granulocytic series.

(*b*) Red Cells and Platelets. The red cells show some variation in size and intensity of staining. A normoblast (*17*) and late erythroblast (*18*) are present in the lower film. In both cases the platelets appear to be increased. There are masses of platelets (*19*) in association with a megakaryocyte nucleus (*20*). The megakaryocyte nucleus (*20*) shows a typical dark rim surrounding masses of chromatin appearing as a wavy structure.

2. *INTERPRETATION.* There is little doubt about the diagnosis when blood films such as those shown in Plate XI are seen. The obvious diagnosis is myelogenous leukemia, because both films are characterized by an extreme increase in the white-cell count and immaturity of the granulocytic series of cells representing all stages. The changes are an order of magnitude greater than occurs in nonleukemic conditions. The abnormalities of the red cells and platelets are also consistent with the complications of leukemia — replacement of the marrow with leukemic tissue. The prognosis of a given case can be estimated in part by an appreciation of the degree of abnormalities in the film.

(*a*) Upper Picture: Chronic Myelogenous Leukemia. In the case with this blood picture, the prognosis is consistent with a chronic process and the patient may be aided considerably by treatment. This prognosis is indicated by the maturity of the granulocytic series. The youngest cells present are the stage of myelocyte B. The presence of basophilic cells in increased numbers is of interest, since basophilic myelocytes are frequently increased in untreated chronic myelogenous leukemia. They may also be relatively increased after radiation therapy, although the absolute number is probably no greater than the pretreatment level [57]. After prolonged radiation therapy, the cells become more and more abortive. This is especially true in the basophils in chronic myelogenous leukemia. Cases in which many basophilic cells have been observed throughout the disease have been called basophilic leukemia [38, 76]. The red cells in this blood film seem quite normal in appearance, but the patient has a significant anemia (see Table 13). The platelets are increased and located in the vicinity of a nuclear fragment of a megakaryocyte. These are frequently seen in the peripheral blood in chronic myelogenous leukemia [193, 195].

(*b*) Lower Picture: Advanced Chronic Myelogenous Leukemia. The prognosis of the patient whose blood film is represented in the lower picture is consistent with an advanced stage of chronic myelogenous leukemia. This is indicated by the marked degree of immaturity of the granulocytic series, which is represented in this instance by the presence of myeloblasts, and by the presence of nucleated red cells. The platelets are markedly increased. A marked increase or a marked decrease in the number of platelets indicates extensive involvement of the bone marrow and is consistent with a bad prognosis.

(*c*) Acute Myelogenous Leukemia. Some cases of leukemia yield a more immature blood film than that shown in either of these pictures. When the predominating cells in the peripheral blood are myeloblasts, the leukemia is considered to be acute or the terminal phase of a chronic leukemia. The myeloblasts in such acute leukemias may be present in many abnormal forms. Some myelocytes may be present with the myeloblasts, an observation which may aid in the identification of the blast form as a myeloblast. Some nucleated red cells are usually present in acute leukemia. The platelets may be markedly decreased in number, large, and abnormal in appearance. Anemia or hemorrhage may be a major cause of death.

(*d*) Subleukemic or Aleukemic Leukemia. If the white-cell count were low, then the interpretation of these blood films would be more difficult. Patients with leukopenia or normal white-cell counts, but with myelocytes or myeloblasts and often nucleated red cells in the blood, may be said to have " subleukemic " myelogenous leukemia. In instances of aleukemic myelogenous leukemia, there may be no, or only a few, abnormal forms of the granulocytic series in the peripheral blood, and a low or normal white-cell count, but there may be nucleated red cells and thrombocytopenia. In these instances of subleukemic or aleukemic leukemia, the diagnosis may be confirmed by bone-marrow puncture or by observing the development of the disease, which may become manifest as leukemia as it advances.

(*e*) Agnogenic Myeloid Metaplasia of the Spleen [147] (Chronic Nonleukemic Myelosis [37, 128], Leuko-erythroblastic Anemia with Myelosclerosis [294], Myelofibrosis [159]). These terms are most frequently used, although in a recent review of the literature Block and Jacobson [25] have mentioned some 25 other designations for this syndrome. In agnogenic myeloid metaplasia, active blood formation takes place in the spleen, liver, or other extramedullary sites. This condition is most easily confused with myelogenous leukemia and the importance of differentiating these two diseases has been pointed out by Jackson, Parker, and Lemon [147], by Hickling [128], and by Block and Jacobson [25]. Myeloid metaplasia may be associated with exposure to industrial solvents such as benzol, and may be preceded by polycythemia [236]. For example, of 15 patients with erythremia reported by Minot and Buckman [194], three developed anemia and a leukemoid blood picture. The sections of the spleen of one of these have been reviewed and showed changes consistent with agnogenic myeloid metaplasia. The description of the blood picture in the cases described by Minot and Buckman [194] and their accompanying plate give an accurate reproduction of the changes in the red and white cells seen in the polycythemic phase of agnogenic myeloid metaplasia. The clinical picture and the hematologic findings vary markedly, especially as the disease progresses. The essential physical finding is progressive and extreme enlargement of the spleen without lymphadenopathy.

The blood film is characterized by marked variation in size and especially in the shape of the red cells, with nucleated red cells. The presence of nucleated red cells occurring when the red-cell count is $4 \times 10^6/\text{mm}^3$ or as high as 6 or $7 \times 10^6/\text{mm}^3$ in cases of polycythemia is a finding of diagnostic importance. In myelogenous leukemia, the red-cell changes early in the disease usually are not so great as in myeloid metaplasia. In myeloid metaplasia, the red cells showed tailed forms, microcytes, and many bizarre forms that are more characteristic of myelophthisic anemia than of any other anemia. Stippled cells, Cabot ring forms, Howell-Jolly bodies, and polychromatophilic cells are found as the disease progresses. Continuing reticulocytosis is characteristic, with occasional cases in the anemic phase showing values as high as 30 percent. A few cases have been observed in which an overwhelming hemolytic anemia has been present [31, 147].

The presence of immature cells of the granulocytic series occurring when the white-cell count is low or normal and the red-cell count is normal or increased is also characteristic. As the disease progresses, more immature cells appear and in some cases the white-cell count may increase to $200 \times 10^3/\text{mm}^3$, making the clinical differentiation from myelogenous leukemia difficult or impossible. The condition may occasionally terminate in leukemia. The disease may be one of prolonged chronicity (20 years) with extreme splenomegaly and with the blood picture described above. In some cases the platelets have been increased, as in myelogenous leukemia, associated with fragments of megakaryocyte nuclei in the film. Platelets may be large and extremely bizarre. In other cases, thrombocytopenic purpura may be the presenting symptom. Splenectomy may be fatal, since active blood formation is taking place in the spleen, although in some instances patients have lived many years [57, 239] following removal of the spleen.

(*f*) Myelophthisic Anemia. In carcinoma arising in the breast, prostate, thyroid, stomach, or kidney, the presence of myelocytes, myeloblasts, and nucleated red cells in the peripheral blood may be the first evidence that metastasis to the bone marrow has occurred [124, 142, 149, 288]. In carcinomatosis there may be a high white-cell count, an increase of myelocytes, occasional myeloblasts, and toxic granulation of the neutrophils. A similar leukemoid response of the myeloid type may be seen in disseminated tuberculosis [142, 287] or when the bone marrow is invaded by lymphoma or leukemic tissue. The presence of nucleated red cells when the red-cell count is above $4 \times 10^6/\text{mm}^3$, and of abnormal cells of the granulocytic series when the white-cell count is normal or slightly increased, should be considered as possible signs of invasion of the bone marrow.

18. PLATE XII. MONOCYTIC LEUKEMIA

1. *DESCRIPTION OF UPPER PICTURE.* The predominating cells in this film are large cells with gray-blue cytoplasm, finely peppered with granules that are concentrated around the periphery. The granules are usually blue-purple but are sometimes azurophilic. These cells are different stages of the monocytic series. As described previously (p. 22), the nucleus of the monocyte is somewhat irregular in outline, is not sharply defined as is the lymphocyte nucleus, and has a lacy, reticular chromatin structure which may have a folded or grooved appearance. As seen in this picture, this lobulation is apparent in the adult monocyte (*6*), in the young monocyte (*7*), and even in the blast (*8*). The nucleus of the mature monocyte (*6*) is indented and the lobes are more striking than in the cells classed as young forms (*7*), which have a round nucleus. This may also be observed in Plate II, in which the monocytes have a typical horseshoe shape. These characteristics should permit differentiation of the monocytic series from the pink-lavender cytoplasm and clumped chromatin nucleus of the neutrophil (*1*) and band form (*2*). The monocyte is nearly always much larger than the neutrophil. In infectious states, abnormally large band forms may be confused with the monocyte. In such instances, the characteristics of the known cells must be compared with those of the unknown. The small lymphocyte (*3*) with clear, light-blue cytoplasm and sharply defined nucleus with condensed chromatin would not be confused with the monocytic series as shown in this film. The red cells are quite uniform in size and shape, but are slightly macrocytic. The platelets are slightly decreased.

2. *DESCRIPTION OF LOWER PICTURE.* In this film the predominating cells are young monocytes (*7*) and blasts (*8*). These are considered monoblasts because they have the same type of folded nucleus as is present in the young and adult monocytes. The three monoblasts (*8a*) with nucleoli represent the youngest cells. The nucleoli are sharply defined areas in the nucleus that take a lighter stain. The nuclear chromatin is slightly more reticular in these blasts than in the myeloblast (Plate XI) or the lymphoblast (Plate XIV). Azurophilic granules may be present in the monoblast and may represent a stage of maturation comparable to the myelocyte A stage in Fig. 4. Azurophilic rods or Auer bodies are present in the cytoplasm of some of these monoblasts (*8b*). It should not be difficult to distinguish the myelocyte with its homogeneous nucleus, sometimes covered with granules (*4*), from the monocyte with its loose reticular nucleus. The histio-

cyte (*5*) in the lower right-hand corner should be observed with care, since this cell is often incorrectly classed as a monocyte. The histiocyte is characterized by the irregular contour of the cell, the spongy, vacuolated cytoplasm which may or may not show active phagocytosis, and the honeycomb structure of the nucleus. The red cells show moderate variation in size. The platelets are definitely reduced, as occurs in most acute leukemias.

3. *INTERPRETATIONS*

(*a*) RÉSUMÉ OF CASES. These blood films are from two patients with monocytic leukemia (A47-30 and A45-310 Mallory Institute of Pathology, Boston City Hospital). The patient whose blood film is shown in the upper picture was a 73-year-old woman who entered the hospital because of anemia (red-cell count, $1.4 \times 10^6/mm^3$; hemoglobin, 5.3 gm/100 ml). She had noted progressive weakness and exertional dyspnea for approximately 1 year. Her diet had been markedly restricted in variety and amount. There were two previous admissions, 7 and 12 years before, with diagnoses of psychoneurosis, malnutrition, and vitamin deficiency. Aspiration of the bone marrow on her last admission showed hyperactivity of granulocytic, monocytic, and erythrocytic series with extremely young red cells. She was first considered to have a nutritional macrocytic anemia and was given liver extract, but her anemia did not respond to therapy. Her white-cell count on admission was $7.1 \times 10^3/mm^3$ with 34 percent of monocytes. The white-cell count increased steadily while under observation to $300 \times 10^3/mm^3$ and the proportion of monocytes increased to 92 percent. Throughout the period of observation the characteristic cells were the large monocytes with gray-blue cytoplasm containing fine scattered blue-purple granules and typical lobulated nuclei with the loose, lacy structure. Young monocytes and monoblasts were present, but the mature forms predominated. The duration of the disease after the diagnosis of leukemia became manifest was only 1 month. Although her presenting symptoms at this admission were those of anemia, presumably related to the leukemia, it is impossible to judge how long the leukemic process had been active.

The blood film shown in the lower picture was from a 41-year-old man with severe anemia, thrombocytopenia, and high white-cell counts. The clinical manifestations at this time were typical of an acute leukemia with a sudden onset 5 days before admission, symptoms of a mild upper-respiratory infection and slight sore throat, headache, and pain in the arms and legs and back. The patient had nosebleeds, petechiae, gastro-intestinal hemorrhage, and bleeding from a rectal fistula. An ischiorectal abscess had been operated upon 5 months previously, but it had not healed properly; no data on the blood film at that time are available. The patient had a rapid downhill course, death occurring after 20 days in the hospital. In contrast to the other case, the white blood cells were chiefly monoblasts and young monocytes.

(*b*) PROGNOSIS IN MONOCYTIC LEUKEMIA. It is difficult to distinguish between acute monocytic leukemia and the terminal phase of chronic monocytic leukemia. Patients have been observed who have shown an increased count of monocytes, largely adult forms, over a period of many months. This has been followed subsequently by clinical manifestations of leukemia and the appearance of increased numbers of young monocytes and monoblasts in the peripheral blood during a terminal "leukemic" period of 2 months [21]. Chronic monocytic leukemia occurs, although definite diagnosis often is not established until the patient has an acute fulminating infection or hemorrhagic manifestations associated with an acute phase of the monocytic leukemia [99]. When the peripheral blood contains monoblasts, the prognosis is poor. However, patients have been observed with mature monocytes in their peripheral blood associated with the symptoms and signs of an acute type of leukemia with gum lesions and hemorrhagic phenomena. The duration of life is influenced in part by the control of the infection with drugs and antibiotics.

(*c*) WHITE-CELL COUNT IN MONOCYTIC LEUKEMIA. The white-cell count varies widely from normal values up to several hundred thousand per cubic millimeter. The predominating cell is the monocyte. A given case may show mature forms as the predominating cell, monoblasts as the characteristic form, or, in most instances, different stages in maturation of the monocyte. As the disease progresses, the type of monocyte may become more and more immature. Young neutrophils and myelocytes may also be seen, but rarely in numbers great enough to cause confusion. Myelocytes may be present in any leukemia or anemia.

(*d*) Auer Bodies. The Auer bodies shown in some of these cells (*8b*) are characteristically seen in acute leukemias [3]. Although they were originally described as occurring in lymphocytes [10], with a better differentiation of the blood cells it is now recognized that they occur in myeloblasts [244], in monoblasts in many cases of monocytic leukemia, in histiocytes or reticulum cells, and in plasma cells [57, 99, 107, 170]. According to Leitner [170], these Auer bodies are crystals of abnormal protein.

(*e*) Anemia. A normocytic anemia (rarely macrocytic as in these two cases) of moderate to severe degree is usually present by the time a diagnosis of monocytic leukemia can be made. Nucleated red cells are often present as one of the characteristics of a myelophthisic anemia.

(*f*) Platelets. The platelet count is usually decreased. This may be manifest, occasionally as a presenting complaint, by hemorrhagic phenomena, as was observed in the patient whose blood film is shown in the lower picture.

4. *MONOCYTIC LEUKEMIA DIFFERENTIATED FROM OTHER LEUKEMIAS.* The separation of monocytic leukemia from other leukemias was first described by Reschad and Schilling-Torgau in 1913 [241]. The hypothesis of Ehrlich [85] that the monocyte was a transition form between the myelocyte and the neutrophil impeded progress in the understanding of this cell. Naegeli [207] and Evans [90] concluded that the monocyte was an independent cell type of myeloid origin. Still further confusion has resulted because the monocyte has not been differentiated by many observers from the histiocyte or reticulum cell. The theories of origin of the monocyte have been confusing. Forkner [99], for example, cites 16 such theories.

Clough [47] reported 22 cases of monocytic leukemia from the literature and one of his own, but did not differentiate the monocyte from the histiocyte. Forkner [99] differentiated acute monocytic leukemia from acute lymphocytic and acute myelogenous leukemia. Other reviews of monocytic leukemia are given by Osgood [219] and by Evans [91].

In the majority of instances, monocytic leukemia need not be confused with either the myelogenous leukemia or the histiocytic leukemia if the type of cell is studied. Although small numbers of myelocytes may be present in a monocytic leukemia, and occasionally there appears to be a " shower " of monocytes in a myelogenous leukemia, these two leukemias are readily distinguishable. It is necessary to evaluate the blood by making more than one observation. For example, Hall and Watkins [115] report a case changing from myelogenous to monocytic leukemia, probably indicating an early myeloid response in a patient with underlying monocytic leukemia.

Watkins and Hall [79, 296] have shown that the Schilling type of monocytic leukemia can be distinguished from the Naegeli form by the morphologic characteristics of the predominant cell and its progenitors and by the histopathologic findings in the hematopoietic tissues. The Schilling type of monocytic leukemia appears to be a separate entity and is called by some leukemic reticulo-endotheliosis (or histiocytic leukemia). A series of leukemia cases have been studied by Belding, Daland, and Parker [21] in which differentiation of histiocytic leukemia from the monocytic leukemia has been possible by hematologic, pathologic, and morphologic studies.

5. *MONOCYTIC RESPONSE — MONOCYTOSIS.* The evaluation of the literature in regard to monocytic responses must also be carefully considered with respect to the type of cell described. The response of histiocytes and clasmatocytes has been termed a " mononuclear " reaction throughout the literature, but is discussed separately (Sec. 19), since these are not cells of the monocytic series.

Monocytes are often increased during the recovery phase of agranulocytosis. They are also increased following acute infection and in pneumonia during the period of resolution of the pulmonary process, in the acute phase of rheumatic fever [57], in some instances of acute inflammation [100], and, in many patients, in the active phase of tuberculosis [23, 187]. Also, the increase in the number of monocytes was found to be of diagnostic importance in selecting, before clinical symptoms developed, the patients who were getting tetrachlorethane poisoning [197]. In conditions associated with monocytosis, the course of the blood findings and the clinical manifestations over a period of time usually serve to differentiate them from monocytic leukemia. Occasionally, the differentiation is obtained only at autopsy, in which the presence or absence of infiltration of the organs by the monocytic leukemia is the criterion for the diagnosis or exclusion of the diagnosis of leukemia.

19. PLATE XIII. HISTIOCYTES IN INFECTIONS AND LEUKEMIA

1. *UPPER PICTURE: BACTERIAL ENDOCARDITIS.*

(*a*) Description. The most striking cells in this picture are the large irregular histiocytes (*6*) with irregular nuclei of varied types, some honeycomblike in structure, some with fine chromatin, some slightly lobulated. Nucleoli may be present (as seen in two cells) even if the cytoplasm is not basophilic. The characteristic cytoplasm may be described as gray-blue, spongy or foamy in structure, vacuolated, and containing phagocytized material such as red cells, white cells, platelets and cellular debris (*8*). These cells sometimes are called macrophages or clasmatocytes. These ameboid histiocytes may be contrasted with the monocytes (*5*) which have a deeper gray-blue cytoplasm containing many granules. The monocytes have lacy, folded, or lobulated nuclei. The large lymphocyte (*4*) has a light-blue cytoplasm and regular nucleus with slightly clumped chromatin. The neutrophils may all be considered as young forms (*2*) and contain toxic granules. The band form (*2a*) in the lower right-hand corner has a large " swollen " nucleus and vacuoles. These characteristics are seen in neutrophils in severe infection and may be evidence of cellular degeneration. The red cells appear to be normal, and the platelets are normal in both number and appearance.

(*b*) Interpretation. The histiocyte that is seen in this condition is usually ameboid in appearance and may show evidence of active phagocytosis. It has been demonstrated that the number of both white cells and histiocytes in the peripheral blood of bacterial endocarditis is much greater in capillary blood taken from the ear lobe than in that from the finger tip, or from the antecubital vein [32, 59, 177, 226, 231]. The number of histiocytes in capillary blood from the ear varies from drop to drop, from hour to hour, and from day to day. No correlation has been found between these fluctuations of the white blood cells and histiocytes in the blood and the clinical manifestations, such as fever and the presence of infarcts or emboli. The concentration of these cells in blood from the ear lobe may be due to local stasis of the cells as a result of the slow circulation of the capillary system in contrast to the arteriovenous anastomoses characteristic of the finger tip. In addition, hyperplastic changes in the endothelium of the ear lobe in bacterial endocarditis [59, 221] probably help trap the large, motile ameboid histiocytes presented by the arterial blood stream.

Differentiation of bacterial endocarditis, with histiocytosis, from leukemia may be difficult. In leukemia the contrast between the white-cell count from the ear lobe and that from the finger or vein is not as striking as it is in bacterial endocarditis. The abnormal cells may be present in the bone-marrow aspiration in leukemia, but are not increased in the bone marrow in bacterial endocarditis.

(*c*) Histiocytes in Infections (Fig. 8, *1* and *2*). The presence of a few histiocytes may occur in the blood early in the course of infections other than bacterial endocarditis. In overwhelming sepsis a terminal shower of histiocytes has been observed [57]. Thirty percent of histiocytes have been seen in a case of meningococcus meningitis (A36-601, Mallory Institute of Pathology) and 52 percent of histiocytes (" ameboid forms of abnormal cells ") were found in a terminal state in a patient with pneumonia. Another patient with peritonitis showed 18 percent of histiocytes just before death (A44-105). There was no evidence of leukemia in these patients. A typhoid fever patient had many ameboid and phagocytic histiocytes in the peripheral blood (Fig. 8, 2) [57].

(*d*) Histiocytes in Anemia (Fig. 8, *4*). Ehrlich [85] probably was the first to describe "mononuclear erythrophagocytosis." Abt [1] observed erythrophagocytosis in a newborn infant with anemia. Histiocytes have been observed many times in the peripheral blood in pernicious anemia. Rowley [250] described a case of anemia characterized by marked phagocytic activity of the histiocytes in the peripheral blood. Histiocytes showing active phagocytosis have frequently been seen in hemolytic anemia [151, 314].

(*e*) Histiocytes in Parasitic Diseases and Rickettsial Diseases. In malaria, histiocytes show active phagocytosis of pigment and products of red-cell destruction in man [249] and in monkey [283]. Foot [98] has described the occurrence of histiocytes in kala azar and in amebiasis. Histiocytes are also seen in the blood in typhus and in Rocky Mountain spotted fever.

(*f*) Histocytes in Letterer-Siwe's Disease. Orchard [218] has reported unusual cells in the peripheral blood of a patient with Letterer-Siwe's syndome. These so-called "haemohistiocytes" were similar to the "reticulum cells" seen in the tissue. Letterer-Siwe's disease, eosinophilic granuloma of the bone and Hand-Schüller-Christian disease are considered by Lichtenstein [172] and others as one entity, "Histiocytosis X," because the proliferating cells in question, derived largely from the reticulo-endothelial cells, display phagocytic activity.

(*g*) Histiocytes in the Storage Diseases. Modified histiocytes are characteristic of Niemann-Pick disease and Gaucher's disease. Although these cells are of diagnostic value in aspiration of spleen and bone marrow, they are only rarely seen in the peripheral blood [285]. Lipoid histiocytosis has been described by Baty [17] in a case of Niemann-Pick disease in which a leukocytosis of from 12.0 to $35.0 \times 10^3/\text{mm}^3$ occurred, with 27 percent of the white cells containing large vacuoles of varying size scattered throughout the abundant pale-blue cytoplasm. The nucleus was somewhat indented and relatively dense. These cells were peroxidase-negative and in supravital stain showed the characteristics of clasmatocytes. Blackfan and Diamond [24] described such cells as phagocytic monocytes or clasmatocytes while Bloom [26] described them as vacuolated monocytes and vacuolated histiocytes.

(*h*) Histiocytes in Virus Infections. The young type of "abnormal lymphocyte" seen in infectious mononucleosis, infectious hepatitis, and chicken pox resembles some of the cells seen in histiocytic leukemia and the terminal phase of Hodgkin's sarcoma. It is possible that this type of cell is produced from the cellular reticulum of the lymph node. Bunting [34] in one of his early papers spoke of the hyperplasia of reticulum cells of the lymph nodes that took place when there was a lymphocytic reaction as a result of antibody production. "Lymphocytic histiocytes" have been described on p. 24.

(*i*) Histiocytes in Allergic Reactions. Some of the young abnormal "lymphocytic cells" seen in serum sickness are irregular cells with basophilic cytoplasm which have the morphological features of histiocytes.

2. *LOWER PICTURE: HISTIOCYTIC LEUKEMIA.*

(*a*) Description. The characteristic cell in this picture is the basophilic leukemic type of histiocyte [21]. This type of histiocyte is definitely larger than the other cells of the blood, and is often more irregular in outline; it varies in size and appearance. The cytoplasm is much deeper blue than the clear blue cytoplasm of the small (*3*) and large (*4*) lymphocyte. The cytoplasm of these histiocytes contains a few scattered granules (sometimes azurophilic) and vacuoles; it even shows phagocytosis of red cells. The chromatin structure of the nucleus of these cells is smooth or finely vacuolated, as in the lower cell (*7*), and not granular as is usual in the blast, or clumped as is characteristic of the lymphocyte. Broken or "basket" cells (*9*) are frequently seen in leukemic bloods and are usually considered to be an index of immature or leukemic cells. The few neutrophils that are seen in such a case are usually young forms (*2*). The platelets are definitely diminished in number. The red cells show slight variation in size.

(*b*) Interpretation. The hematologic observations for Plate XIII are given in Table 15. This picture of a blood film was from a patient with histiocytic leukemia, one of the series published by Belding and associates [21] in which a clinical summary of this patient (Case 4) and a chart showing the hematologic findings during the course of the disease (Fig. 4) are given.

The diagnosis of histiocytic leukemia is first suggested by the appearance in the peripheral blood of large, irregular cells which do not conform to the characteristics of the granulocytic, monocytic, lymphocytic, or plasma-cell series. This may best be seen by comparing the cells in Plate XIII with the cells of the granulocytic series in Plate XI, the monocytic series in Plate XII, the lymphocytic series in Plate XIV and the plasma-cell series in Plate XV. Not only are these cells different from those of the regular series, but the type of cell varies markedly in a given blood sample and is quite distinctive in different cases. The variation in size and nuclear structure is quite obvious in Plate XIII. In this picture the contrast between the lymphocytes, monocytes, and neutrophils is striking. In this particular case the cytoplasm is deeply basophilic, but the structure of the nucleus is not granular like a blast and does not show nucleoli. Phagocytosis of red cells, as shown in Plate XIII, was seen in the peripheral blood, in the bone-marrow aspirations, and in the fixed tissues. In some cases the cells may have a characteristic " blast nucleus," with granular chromatin and nucleoli, but still have a light cytoplasm which is not as basophilic as would be expected in a " blast." The cells are more often confused with lymphocytes or blasts than with monocytes. The histiocytes, as well as lymphocytes and blasts, show a negative peroxidase reaction, while the monocytes are usually peroxidase-positive, as are all the cells of the granulocytic series with the exception of the blasts.

The white-cell count in the blood film shown in Plate XIII is high ($28.9 \times 10^3/mm^3$), but many of the cases studied [21] have shown a normal or low count. When the white-cell count is below $3.0 \times 10^3/mm^3$, differential cell counts are more difficult and the few abnormal forms may easily be classified as atypical lymphocytes. However, these irregular basophilic cells may be the important cells which give the clue that the diagnosis may be histiocytic leukemia. When the white-cell count is low, a buffy coat of the white cells should be studied for the identification of the blast cells. Bone-marrow aspirations should also be obtained in such cases. A biopsy of the bone marrow, lymph node, or skin lesions, which are often present, should be made for confirmation of the diagnosis.

(*c*) Histiocytic Leukemia in the Literature. The literature on histiocytic leukemia is confused because many of the early investigators failed to distinguish the histiocyte from the monocyte. Downey [79, 80] differentiated the Schilling type of monocytic leukemia (histiocytic) from the Naegeli type of monocytic leukemia (monocytic). Later, Montgomery and Watkins [200], and Watkins and Hall [296] reviewed some of the clinical and hematologic differences between these two types of leukemia. There are many case reports of histiocytic leukemia in the literature, but this condition has been designated by a variety of terms, such as " histioleukemia " [199], " reticulosis " [138], " aleukemic reticulosis " [64], " leukemic reticulo-endotheliosis " [80, 97], and " clasmatocytic leukemia " [103]; in addition there are those cases which are included within the broad term " monocytic leukemia " [63, 72].

(*d*) Histiocytes in Reticulum-Cell Sarcoma and Hodgkin's Sarcoma (Fig. 8, *3* and *5*). Although the blood findings in Hodgkin's disease are not considered to be diagnostic [145], there are cases of Hodgkin's sarcoma and reticulum-cell sarcoma in which both the ameboid or phagocytic type of histiocyte and the basophilic or leukemic histiocyte have been seen in the peripheral blood. There may be leukopenia, normal white-cell count, or increased white-cell count due to the increase of abnormal cells (leukemic histiocytes). The type of cell seen in some of these cases is quite similar to those in histiocytic leukemia (Plate XIII). Such a patient (P. H. 19588), in whom a leukemic blood picture was present during the last hospital admission, the white-cell count varying from 4.0 to $2.0 \times 10^3/mm^3$, was reported by Merrill and Jackson [189]. The abnormal cells, which varied from 2 to 36 percent, were large irregular forms with deep-blue cytoplasm and nuclei of homogeneous chromatin with nucleoli. These were considered to be histiocytes. Other cases have been observed with histiocytes of various types appearing repeatedly in the film of the peripheral blood [57]. These may be seen more readily if the blood films are obtained from the ear lobe, as the large cells are often more concentrated in this area in which the capillary circulation may be rather sluggish [59]. When abnormal cells of this type appear in the peripheral blood, the bone-marrow aspiration may show masses of these leukemic histiocytes. Biopsy of the lymph nodes, skin lesions, if present, or bone marrow is usually indicated to confirm the diagnosis in such cases.

In the review by Dameshek [64] a relation between " aleukemic reticulosis " and Hodgkin's disease was suggested. Marchal and Bargeton [184] report that Hodgkin's sarcoma may show a terminal " monocytosis "; these monocytes are presumably histiocytes.

20. PLATE XIV. LYMPHOCYTIC LEUKEMIA

1. *UPPER PICTURE: CHRONIC LYMPHOCYTIC LEUKEMIA.*

(*a*) DESCRIPTION. The predominating cell in this film is the mature lymphocyte with its clear-blue cytoplasm. The nucleus of the lymphocyte (*3*) is rather sharply defined and contains densely clumped chromatin, whereas the nucleus in the monocyte (*2*) is irregular, sometimes horseshoe-shaped, and has a delicate lacy structure or fine network.

The mature lymphocyte is divided into two types according to size. The small lymphocyte (*3*) has a nucleus about the size of a red cell and a relatively small amount of cytoplasm. The large lymphocyte (*4*) has a nucleus larger than the red cell and usually has abundant cytoplasm. The structure of the nucleus is similar to that of the small lymphocyte, but often is not so densely clumped. The cytoplasm is a clear blue, the lightest blue of any of the blood cells, and occasionally contains a few scattered red-purple granules, and rarely some blue granules.

Broken cells (*7*) are common in films of leukemic blood and are not included in the differential count of white cells because the cell type cannot usually be identified. The red cells show slightly more than normal variation in size. The number of platelets is slightly decreased.

(*b*) INTERPRETATION. This picture is characteristic of the blood film seen in chronic lymphocytic leukemia. Here the predominating cell is the small lymphocyte (*3*) (see p. 19). Sometimes the nuclear chromatin is more densely clumped than normal, giving the appearance of plasma cells. Such cells can usually be differentiated from plasma cells by the fact that the lymphocyte cytoplasm is a clear light blue compared to the green-blue of the plasma cell (see Plate XV). Occasionally vacuoles or fenestrations of the nucleus will simulate nucleoli, but true nucleoli are usually seen in young forms with deep basophilic cytoplasm. The nucleus is usually round, although certain cases of leukemia have been observed in which the nuclei have deep indentations [57].

The degree of anemia varies from none to severe myelophthisic forms with variable degrees of thrombocytopenia.

Chronic lymphocytic leukemia may be discovered by accident and the patient may live many years. Accordingly, the identification of mature lymphocytes by careful study of the blood film is an aid in establishing the prognosis of the patient.

2. *LOWER PICTURE: ACUTE LYMPHOCYTIC LEUKEMIA.*

(*a*) DESCRIPTION. The cells in this film are more immature than those shown in the upper picture. The predominating cell types are the young lymphocyte (*5*) and the lymphoblast (*6*). The nucleus of the young lymphocyte does not stain so intensely as the nucleus in the small or large lymphocytes, and the chromatin is not so densely packed. The nucleus is large and occupies most of the cell, leaving only a small rim of deep-blue cytoplasm. The nucleus of the lymphoblast has a red-purple, finely granular chromatin structure and stains less intensely than any of the more mature forms. Three of the lymphoblasts in this film have nucleoli. The cytoplasm of the lymphoblast is not abundant and stains a deep blue similar to that of the young lymphocyte. The lymphoblast (*6*) may be contrasted with the small (*3*) and large lymphocytes (*4*) that are present in the film. Broken cells (*7*) or "smudges" are seen in increased numbers in acute leukemias and are noted but not included in the differential count of white cells.

The red cells show greater variation in size and shape in the lower picture than in the upper picture, and there is a marked decrease in the number of platelets, a frequent finding in acute leukemia.

(*b*) Interpretation. This picture may be compared with the upper picture showing the chronic form of the disease. This might be either an acute leukemia or the terminal stage of a chronic form. The presence of lymphoblasts, changes in the red cells associated with the anemia, and thrombocytopenia, as shown in this film, are diagnostic points that give a serious prognosis for the patient. This patient lived only 3 weeks after this examination of his blood was made.

Anemia in these leukemias may be the result of acute or chronic blood loss because of the thrombocytopenia, or it may be a myelophthisic anemia showing nucleated red cells and myelocytes resulting from infiltration of the bone marrow.

21. PLATE XV. PLASMA-CELL LEUKEMIA

1. *DESCRIPTION OF UPPER PICTURE.* The predominating cells in this blood film are the mature plasma cells [190] which are characterized by an elongated or oval shape with an eccentric nucleus (*5*) and, in some, by a perinuclear clear area. The cytoplasm is a characteristic gray green-blue with a foamy or spongy structure, sometimes containing vacuoles, and showing ragged edges. This cytoplasm is quite different from the clear-blue cytoplasm of the lymphocyte (*2*). The mature plasma cell has a characteristic nucleus with wedges of chromatin that are distinctly separated, in contrast to the more compact nuclear structure of the lymphocyte. The cell with the double nucleus is a plasma cell in division. The presence of dividing cells suggests the possibility of a neoplastic disease involving the plasma cell, such as plasmacytoma (myeloma) or plasma-cell leukemia. The plasma cell is easily confused with the erythroblast (*11*), which may have a similar nucleus but has a gray-blue, homogeneous cytoplasm containing no vacuoles and a cell outline that is smooth and not ragged.

The red cells show very little variation in size and shape. However, they appear in groups or in moderate rouleaux (*9a*), which are associated with hyperglobulinemia in many but not all cases. The observation of rouleaux in a thin film is indicative of increased concentrations of fibrinogen or serum globulins.

The platelets are normal in morphology, but appear slightly decreased in number.

2. *DESCRIPTION OF LOWER PICTURE.* The types of plasma cells in this picture are more varied than in the upper picture. Since many stages of plasma cells are represented, these cells are more difficult to classify. Two mature forms are shown (*5*) with characteristic eccentric nuclei, oval shape, irregular outline, and a purple (rather than gray green-blue) reaction of the cytoplasm (*5b* and *5c*). The purple color of these cells appears to arise from a mixture of color resulting from acidophilic material and basophilic material. In one of these cells (*5c*), acidophilic material appears as globules called Russell bodies [190, 230].

The young plasma cells (*6*) have a gray green-blue cytoplasm with some vacuolated areas, but the nuclear structure is finer than that of the mature cells. These cells are exceedingly difficult to distinguish from the large lymphocyte (*3*), in which the cytoplasm is a clear blue. The characteristic gray green-blue or muddy blue of the immature plasmacyte aids in its identification. Also, these cells are usually seen in association with some mature forms.

There are two blast forms present; one is the youngest form of the plasmacytic series (*7*) and has the characteristic blue cytoplasm and vacuoles. The other blast (*8*) may be considered an unidentified blast form or a stem cell. The stem cell is usually much larger than the other blasts and has basophilic cytoplasm staining a much deeper blue than that of blast forms. The nucleus is finely granular, stains less intensely than the cytoplasm, and contains several nucleoli which are large and distinct. Stem cells may be seen in any leukemic blood or severe infection that demands young cells from the hematopoietic tissues. Sometimes a leukemia characterized by young cells of this type is called a stem-cell leukemia.

This film also shows a normal monocyte (*4*) and a normoblast (*10*). The red cells show the rouleau formation that is characteristic of the diseases with high globulin concentrations.

3. *INTERPRETATION OF BOTH PICTURES.*

(*a*) Peripheral Blood. These pictures represent two cases of plasma-cell leukemia, which is a rare condition [203, 227]. Diagnosis is not difficult when the cells are typical and mature, as in the upper picture. The problem is much greater in the lower picture, where many stages of plasma-cell development are seen. By carefully studying these cells, the same characteristic cytoplasm (gray green-blue, vacuolated, or spongy) can be seen. Plasma-cell leukemia is considered as the leukemic phase of plasmocytoma (multiple myeloma) [146]. In the blood of both patients shown in Plate XV there was a myelophthisic anemia.

(*b*) Bone-Marrow Studies in Plasmocytoma. A study of bone-marrow aspirations in multiple myeloma may give varied pictures in different cases. In some instances, the mature plasma cell, such as is seen in the upper picture, predominates, while in others the young plasma cell or the plasmablast may predominate. These young forms of plasma cells have the same characteristics as the so-called myeloma cell [18, 19, 74, 201]. In some cases, the bone marrow has the variety of cells shown in the lower picture of plasma-cell leukemia.

(*c*) Plasma Cells in Other Conditions. Cells of the plasmacytic series may appear in the bone marrow and peripheral blood in instances of hyperplasia of the hematopoietic system and in many infections such as measles, infectious mononucleosis, chicken pox [132], overwhelming sepsis, and serum sickness [158], and in the recovery phase of agranulocytosis [54, 170].

The Türk irritation form, reported by many observers in infectious diseases, is probably a cell of the plasmacytic series.

(*d*) Histochemistry. The periodic acid Schiff method of McManus and Hotchkiss has been used, together with other techniques, to investigate the cytochemistry of plasma cells [230]. Evidence is presented to show that the cytoplasm of human plasma cells contains mucoprotein [230], which is a polysaccharide-containing globulin. If the function of the plasma cell is to produce mucoproteins, then the formation of Russell bodies may represent a disorder due to overstimulation or overproduction. The presence of mucoprotein in the cytoplasm and Russell bodies may account for their similarity in staining, as shown by the acidophilic cytoplasm and the Russell bodies in cells *5b* and *5c*.

(*e*) Anemia. Anemia is a frequent complication of the infiltration of bone marrow by plasma cells and is usually myelophthisic.

22. PLATE XVI. INFECTIOUS MONONUCLEOSIS

1. *DESCRIPTION OF UPPER PICTURE.* The first impression when one looks at a blood film like that shown in the upper picture is that of a lymphocytosis. On more careful study, it becomes a question whether these cells are lymphocytes or monocytes, for they have many abnormal features. The predominating cell is an abnormal or atypical lymphocyte (*4*) showing the following characteristics: large size, being as large as or larger than the monocyte (*3*) shown in the same field; irregular shape of the cytoplasm; irregular shape of the nucleus; and clear-blue cytoplasm which varies in intensity of staining. The periphery appears deeper blue than other areas, as if the cytoplasm were compressed. There may be red or purple granules present in the cytoplasm, but these are scattered and not "peppered" through the cytoplasm, as in the normal monocyte (*3*). In the atypical lymphocytes, the chromatin of the nucleus is not so condensed as

in the small lymphocyte, but there may be aggregations of chromatin around the edge or in clumps through the nucleus. The chromatin is less condensed than in the small lymphocyte (*2*), but is not as lacy or reticular in structure as in the monocyte. The atypical lymphocytes apparently are more fragile than normal white cells and may appear as fragmented forms in fixed preparations. The group of atypical lymphocytes in the upper drawing corresponds to the Type II described by Downey [82] and to those illustrated in the report of Baldridge, Rohner, and Hansmann [11].

The red cells and platelets in this film are normal.

2. *DESCRIPTION OF LOWER PICTURE.* The blood film represented here is a real problem in diagnosis, because practically all the white cells are abnormal. A careful study shows that there is one normal small lymphocyte (*2*) and a blast form (*7*) with fine granular chromatin structure of the nucleus and deep-blue cytoplasm. The fact that most of the cells are immature, as indicated by their deep-blue cytoplasm, makes classification more difficult. From the characteristics of these cells alone, differentiation between the monocytic series and lymphocytic series cannot be made with certainty. In fact, these cells are similar to some histiocytes and may be histiocytes from lymphatic tissue. However, the occurrence of immature forms (*6*) together with the cells containing vacuolated cytoplasm (*5*) suggests hyperplasia of lymphoid tissue due to infectious mononucleosis. These abnormal young forms, which usually are called immature atypical lymphocytes, are similar to those described by Downey as Type III and the vacuolated forms correspond to Downey's Type I [82].

Plasma cells (*8*) are also common when there is a lymphoid hyperplasia. The plasma cell shown here is also atypical in that the nucleus is not eccentric.

The platelets appear to be normal and the red cells show slight variation in size.

3. *INTERPRETATION OF BOTH PICTURES.*

(*a*) Morphology of White Cells in Infectious Mononucleosis. The blood pictures represented here are from two different patients with infectious mononucleosis. These changes are also seen in different stages of the disease in the same patient. It is difficult, however, to correlate the degree of immaturity of the white cells seen in the blood film with the severity of the illness of the patient or with the phase of disease. The pictures are characterized by pathologic mononuclear cells that do not conform to normal stages in development of either the monocytic or the lymphocytic series. The study of these cells by means of supravital technic [102, 166, 304] has led to the conclusion that they belong to the lymphocytic series. Some of the immature forms have nucleoli, but the nucleus is more irregular in shape and the chromatin is more clumped than in the typical lymphoblasts. The cells in this plate should be carefully compared with those of Plates XII, XIII, XIV, and XV to appreciate the abnormal features of these cells.

The review by Bernstein [22] gives many important facts about the course of the disease. These abnormal cells may exist early in the disease, but typically they appear within the first 4 or 5 days of illness and rapidly reach a maximum within a week or 10 days. The proportion of " mononuclear " atypical lymphocytes in the cases studied varied from 40 to 90 percent. Some of these abnormal forms may persist for 9 or 10 months after the patient has recovered from clinical signs of the disease.

(*b*) White-Cell Count. The white-cell count may show a marked leukopenia during the first week, but a leukocytosis characterized by atypical and normal lymphocytes is the rule. In 65 cases studied, Bernstein found that 86 percent of the white-cell counts were between 8.0 and 20.0 $\times$ $10^3/mm^3$ [22]. In a few instances, the white-cell counts exceeded 40.0 $\times$ $10^3/mm^3$.

(*c*) Forms of White Cells Other than Atypical Lymphocytes. The changes in the blood picture should be followed during the course of the disease, as in all infections. The number of eosinophils is decreased during the acute phase, as in many infections, but increases during convalescence. Myelocytes may be present in patients who are severely ill. The neutrophils are characterized by immature forms (bands), often with toxic granulation.

(*d*) Red Cells and Platelets. It is important

to emphasize that the red cells in uncomplicated infectious mononucleosis are normal. This is in contrast to the frequent occurrence of anemia as a complication of leukemia. However, the blood picture of infectious mononucleosis may be superimposed on that of any other condition, including diseases involving red cells, such as hypochromic anemia, hemolytic jaundice, anemia due to hemorrhage, or dietary deficiency. Stippled cells have been seen in some cases.

The platelets are usually normal in infectious mononucleosis. However, a few cases with thrombocytopenia have been reported [22].

(*e*) Heterophile Antibody. The Paul-Bunnell test for heterophile antibody is positive in most cases of infectious mononucleosis at some time during the course of the disease. The heterophile antibody in this disease is not absorbed by guinea-pig kidney, a test that is highly specific for infectious mononucleosis [116, 228].

(*f*) General Features of Infectious Mononucleosis. Infectious mononucleosis may be associated with abnormalities of almost any system or organ, thus giving protean manifestations. The outstanding features of " glandular fever " are fever, lymphadenopathy, sore throat, malaise, headache, and gastro-intestinal symptoms. There is usually a mild or moderate degree of hepatitis.

(*g*) Differentiation from Leukemia. Infectious mononucleosis is often diagnosed as leukemia, because of the bizarre forms and immaturity of the white blood cells. In the leukemias, however, anemia and thrombocytopenia usually are evident by the time the patient seeks medical attention. The heterophile test is uniformly negative in leukemia. In infectious mononucleosis, anemia and thrombocytopenia are not characteristic features of the disease. The differentiation of the cell types has been discussed here and in the description of Plate XIV.

(*h*) Atypical Lymphocytes in Conditions Other than Infectious Mononucleosis. Atypical lymphocytes similar to the varieties seen in infectious mononucleosis are found in a number of other conditions. In some cases the clinical features of the illness are sufficient to make a differential diagnosis, in some the use of the heterophile test with differential absorption of the antibodies is necessary to differentiate infectious mononucleosis from conditions giving a similar blood picture. Young lymphocytes and all stages of plasma cells may be seen in increased numbers in many of these conditions in which the atypical lymphocytes appear.

Infectious hepatitis. An excellent description of the abnormal lymphocytes in infectious (epidemic) jaundice is reported by Minot and Jones [196] and has been confirmed by more recent studies [12, 122]. Although the white-cell count is seldom above normal and often shows leukopenia [286], there is a relative lymphocytosis which frequently shows atypical lymphocytes, young lymphocytes, and cells of the plasmacytic series. The heterophile test in infectious (epidemic) hepatitis is uniformly negative. This is of importance because most patients with infectious mononucleosis have hepatitis which may not be demonstrable clinically but is occasionally associated with jaundice.

Serum sickness. The abnormal lymphocytes in serum sickness may be indistinguishable from those of infectious mononucleosis. The atypical forms include irregularly shaped, vacuolated, and immature lymphocytes which may constitute as many as 30 percent of the white cells. Plasma cells of all stages also appear in increased numbers. The unabsorbed serum may show a high concentration of heterophile antibody. However, the heterophile antibody (Forssman antibody) of serum sickness is completely absorbed by guinea-pig kidney, which does not remove the heterophile antibody of infectious mononucleosis [116].

Chicken pox. In an excellent study of the blood picture in 56 patients with varicella, Holbrook [132] has shown that there is an increase of lymphocytes during the leukopenic phase of the disease. During this stage there is an increase of young lymphocytes, lymphoblasts, and abnormal forms, some showing mitotic figures. An increase in plasma cells also occurred in 50 percent of the cases, to levels as high as 6 or 8 percent in some instances. In another study [57], a case has been observed with the following percentages of cells in the differential count: lymphocytes, 27; young lymphocytes, 17; irregular lymphocytes, 5; vacuolated lymphocytes, 2; and in addition, cells of the plasmacytic series, 7.

Primary atypical pneumonia. A study of the blood picture in 28 cases of virus pneumonia, including 126 white-cell counts, showed that 68 counts (54 percent) were within the normal range (5 to $10 \times 10^3/\text{mm}^3$); 5 counts were under $5 \times 10^3/\text{mm}^3$ and 53 counts were over $10 \times 10^3/\text{mm}^3$ [57]. Many of these higher counts occurred during the third and fourth weeks of the disease. A greater number of lymphocytes is found early in the disease than is seen in pneumococcus pneumonia. There was a slight to moderate increase of young and irregular lymphocytes, such as is seen in infectious mononucleosis, during this lymphoid response. One patient showed up to 9 percent and another 5 percent of these cells. Plasma cells were occasionally seen.

Other conditions. Abnormal lymphocytes may be present in normal individuals, especially children, in hyperthyroidism, typhoid fever, and infections other than the virus diseases. These observations suggest that the appearance of atypical lymphocytes is of no single diagnostic significance but apparently indicates a particular type of response of lymphocytic tissue.

(*i*) LYMPHOCYTOSIS AND LEUKEMOID REACTIONS OF LYMPHOCYTIC TYPE. Lymphocytosis, either absolute or relative, is seen in many virus infections at some stage in the disease, and in other infectious diseases during the period of recovery. The atypical cells, characteristic of infectious mononucleosis, are not usually present.

Relative lymphocytosis is the rule in conditions associated with neutropenia, for example, pernicious anemia, aplastic anemia, agranulocytosis, overwhelming sepsis, influenza, typhoid fever, typhus fever, malaria, measles, and mumps.

Some of the conditions showing an absolute lymphocytosis are acute infectious lymphocytosis of unknown etiology [8, 270], thyrotoxicosis [57, 127, 188], German measles (rubella) [178], whooping cough, typhoid fever, and congenital syphilis [11]. Lymphocytosis simulating lymphocytic leukemia has been reported in two cases of miliary tuberculosis [104], in a case of adenocarcinoma of the sigmoid [238], and in a patient with carcinoma of the breast with metastasis to lungs and spleen [156] (A49-60, Mallory Institute of Pathology).

REFERENCES

1. Abt, A. F., "Mononuclear erythrophagocytosis in the blood of a newborn infant," *Am. J. Dis. Child.* **42**, 1364–1371 (1931).
2. Abt, A. F., and Bloom, W., "Essential lipoid histiocytosis (type Niemann-Pick). A congenital disturbance in lipoid metabolism in infants associated with a splenohepatomegaly," *J. A. M. A.* **90**, 2076–2080 (1928).
3. Ackerman, G. A., "Microscopic and histochemical studies on the Auer bodies in leukemic cells," *Blood* **5**, 847–863 (1950).
4. Aksoy, M., Lehmann, H., and Lie-Injo, L. E., "The recognition of haemoglobins A_2 and E," *Lancet* **1**, 792–793 (1957).
5. Alder, A., "Ueber morphologische Veränderungen anden weissen Blutkörperchen bei Infektionskrankheiten," *Schweiz. med. Wchnschr.* **19**, 440–442 (1921).
6. Allison, A. C., "Notation for hemoglobin types and genes controlling their syndromes," *Science* **122**, 640 (1955).
7. Armand-Delille, P. F., Hurst, A. R., and Sorapure, V. E., "Familial eosinophilia," *Guy's Hosp. Rep.* **80**, 248–252 (1930).
8. Arneil, G. C., and Riley, I. D., "Acute infectious lymphocytosis," *Quart. J. Med.* (n.s.) **21**, 285–290 (1952).
9. Arneth, J., "Die neutrophilen Leukozyten bei Infektionskrankheiten," *Deutsche med. Wchnschr.* **30**, 54–56 (1904).
10. Auer, J., "Some hitherto undescribed structures in the large lymphocytes of a case of acute leukemia," *Am. J. M. Sc.* **131**, 1002–1015 (1906).
11. Baldridge, C. W., Rohner, F. J., and Hansmann, G. H., "Glandular fever (infectious mononucleosis)," *Arch. Int. Med.* **38**, 413–448 (1926).
12. Barker, H. M., Capps, R. B., and Allen, F. W., "Acute infectious hepatitis in the Mediterranean theater," *J. A. M. A.* **128**, 997–1003 (1945).
13. Barnett, C. W., "Unavoidable error in differential count of leukocytes of blood," *J. Clin. Investigation* **12**, 77–85 (1933).
14. Barret, A. M., "A special form of erythrocyte possessing increased resistance to hypotonic saline," *J. Path. & Bact.* **46**, 603–618 (1938).
15. Bassen, F. A., and Kornzweig, A. L., "Malformation of the erythrocytes in a case of atypical retinitis pigmentosa," *Blood* **5**, 381–387 (1950).
16. Battle, J. D., Jr., and Lewis, L. A., "Sickle cell trait and thalassemia minor," *Clin. Research Proc.* **1**, 3 (1953).
17. Baty, J. M., "Lipoid histiocytosis (Niemann's disease)," *Am. J. Dis. Child.* **39**, 573–585 (1930).
18. Bayrd, E. D., "The bone marrow on sternal aspiration in multiple myeloma," *Blood* **3**, 987–1018 (1948).
19. Bayrd, E. D., and Heck, F. J., "Multiple myeloma. A review of eighty-three proved cases," *J. A. M. A.* **133**, 147–157 (1947).
20. Begemann, N. H., and Campagne, A. V., "Homozygous form of Pelger-Huët's nuclear anomaly in man," *Acta haemat.* **7**, 295–303 (1952).
21. Belding, H. W., Daland, G. A., and Parker, F., Jr., "Histiocytic and monocytic leukemia, a clinical, hematological and pathological differentiation," *Cancer* **8**, 237–252 (1955).
22. Bernstein, A., "Infectious mononucleosis," *Medicine* **19**, 85–159, 1940.
23. Blackfan, K. D., and Diamond, L. K., "The monocyte in active tuberculosis. Supravital studies of the blood," *Am. J. Dis. Child.* **37**, 233–243 (1929).
24. Blackfan, K. D., Diamond, L. K., and Leister, C. M., *Atlas of the blood in children* (The Commonwealth Fund, New York, 1944), Plate 49.
25. Block, M., and Jacobson, L. O., "Myeloid metaplasia," *J. A. M. A.* **143**, 1390–1396 (1950).
26. Bloom, W., "The histogenesis of essential lipoid histiocytosis (Niemann-Pick's disease)," *Arch. Path.* **6**, 827–859 (1928).
27. Boros, J. von, "Die Behandlung der Anämien," *Ergebn. d. inn Med. u. Kinderh* **42**, 635–740 (1932).
28. Boveri, R. M., "Howell Jolly bodies and splenic atrophy," *Guy's Hosp. Rep.* **91**, 81–90 (1942).
29. Bradford, W. L., and Dye, J., "Observations on the morphology of the erythrocytes in Mediterranean disease — thalassemia (erythroblastic anemia of Cooley)," *J. Pediat.* **9**, 312–317 (1936).
30. Brecher, G., and Cronkite, E. P., "Morphology and enumeration of human blood platelets," *J. Applied Physiol.* **3**, 365–377 (1950).
31. Brewster, H. H., and Wollenman, O. J., "Myeloid metaplasia of the spleen with acute hemolytic anemia," *New England J. Med.* **227**, 822–825 (1942).
32. Broustet, P., Saric, Léger, Bergaud, A., and Borchard, Mlle., "Cellules endothélioides hémohistioblastiques et variation de la formule du sang capillaire et du sang veineux dans la maladie d'Osler," *Arch. d. mal. du coeur* **39**, 294–300 (1946).
33. Buckman, T. E., "Splenomegaly in infants and children," *M. Clin. North America* **8**, 1551–1575 (1925).
34. Bunting, C. H., "Cell reactions in resistance and immunity," *Wisconsin M. J.* **24**, 305–308 (1925).
35. Cabot, R. C., "Ring bodies (nuclear remnants) in anemic blood," *J. M. Research* **4**, 15–18 (1903).
36. Caminopetros, J., "Recherches sur l'anemie erythroblastique infantile, des peuple de la Méditerranée orientale," *Ann. de méd.* **43**, 104–125 (1938)
37. Carpenter, G., and Flory, C. M., "Chronic nonleukemic myelosis, report of a case with megakaryocytic myeloid splenomegaly, leukoerythroblas-

tic anemia, generalized osteosclerosis and myelofibrosis," *Arch. Int. Med.* **67**, 489–508 (1941).

38. Casey, A. E., Nettles, T. E., and Hidden, E. H., "Basophilic leukemia," *South. M. J.* **39**, 325–332 (1946).
39. Castle, W. B., "Disorders of the blood," Chap. 28 in Sodeman, W. A., *Pathologic physiology: Mechanisms of disease* (W. B. Saunders, Philadelphia, 1956).
40. Castle, W. B., and Daland, G. A., "Susceptibility of mammalian erythrocytes to hemolysis with hypotonic solutions," *Arch. Int. Med.* **60**, 949–966 (1937).
41. Chernoff, A. I., "The human hemoglobins in health and disease," *New England J. Med.* **253**, 322–331, 365–374, 416–423 (1955).
42. Chernoff, A. I., Minnich, V., and Chongcharoensuk, S., "Hemoglobin E, a hereditary abnormality of human hemoglobin," *Science* **120**, 605–606 (1954).
43. Chernoff, A. I., Minnich, V., Chongcharoensuk, S., Na Nakorn, S., and Chernoff, R., "Clinical, hematological and genetic studies of hemoglobin E," *J. Lab. & Clin. Med.* **44**, 780–781 (1954).
44. Chernoff, A. I., and Singer, K., "Studies on abnormal hemoglobins. IV. Persistance of fetal hemoglobin in the erythrocytes of normal children," *Pediat.* **9**, 469–474 (1952).
45. Choremis, C., and Zannos, L., "Microdrepanocytic disease in Greece," *Blood* **12**, 454–460 (1957).
46. Claudon, D. B., and Holbrook, A. A., "Fatal aplastic anemia associated with chloramphenicol (chloromycetin) therapy, report of 2 cases," *J. A. M. A.* **149**, 912–914 (1952).
47. Clough, P. W., "Monocytic leukemia," *Bull. Johns Hopkins Hosp.* **51**, 148–177 (1932).
48. "Committee for clarification of the nomenclature of cells and diseases of the blood and blood-forming organs; condensation of first two reports," *Blood* **4**, 89–96 (1949).
49. Conn, H. J., *Biological stains, a handbook on the nature and use of the dyes employed in the biological laboratory* (Biotech. Publications, Geneva, N.Y., ed. 5, 1946).
50. Conn, H. O., "Sickle-cell trait and splenic infarction associated with high-altitude flying," *New England J. Med.* **251**, 417–420 (1954).
51. Cooley, T. B., and Lee, P., "The rôle of erythrocyte fragmentation in the genesis of anemia," *J. Pediat.* **3**, 55–63, 1933.
52. Coventry, W. D., "Cyclic neutropenia, report of a case treated by spenectomy," *J. A. M. A.* **153**, 28–31 (1925).
53. Cunningham, R. S., Sabin, F. R., and Doan, C. A., *The development of leucocytes, lymphocytes, and monocytes from a specific stem-cell in adult tissues,* Carnegie Institution of Washington, Pub. No. 361 (1925), p. 227 (Contributions to embryology, No. 84).
54. Custer, R. P., *Atlas of blood and bone marrow* (W. B. Saunders, Philadelphia, 1949).
55. Dacie, J. V., *The haemolytic anaemias, congenital and acquired* (Grune & Stratton, New York, 1954).
56. Dacie, J. V., and White, J. D., "Erythropoiesis with particular reference to its study by biopsy of human bone marrow: a review," *J. Clin. Path.* **2**, 1–32 (1949).
57. Daland, G. A., personal observations.
58. Daland, G. A., and Castle, W. B., A simple and rapid method for demonstrating sickling of the red blood cells: the use of reducing agents, *J. Lab. & Clin. Med.* **33**, 1082–1088 (1948).
59. Daland, G. A., Gottlieb, L., Wallerstein, R. O., and Castle, W. B., "Hematologic observations in bacterial endocarditis: especially the prevalence of histiocytes and the elevation and the variation of the white cell count in blood from the ear lobe," *J. Lab. & Clin. Med.* **48**, 827–845 (1956).
60. Daland, G. A., and Hanson, M. L., unpublished data.
61. Daland, G. A., Heath, C. W., and Minot, G. R., "Differentiation of pernicious anemia and certain other macrocytic anemias by the distribution of red blood cell diameters," *Blood* **1**, 67–75 (1946).
62. Daland, G. A., and Strauss, M. B., "The genetic relation and clinical differentiation of Cooley's anemia and Cooley's trait," *Blood* **3**, 438–448 (1948).
63. Dameshek, W., "Acute monocytic (histiocytic) leukemia: review of the literature and case reports," *Arch. Int. Med.* **46**, 718–740 (1930).
64. Dameshek, W., "Proliferative diseases of the reticulo-endothelial system: aleukemic reticulosis," *Folia haemat.* **49**, 64–85 (1933).
65. Dameshek, W., "'Target cell' anemia, anerythroblastic type of Cooley's erythroblastic anemia," *Am. J. M. Sc.* **200**, 445–454 (1940).
66. Dameshek, W., "Familial Mediterranean target-oval cell syndromes," *Am. J. M. Sc.* **205**, 643–660 (1943).
67. Dameshek, W., Henstell, H. H., and Valentine, E. H., "The comparative value and the limitations of the trephine and puncture method for biopsy of the sternal bone marrow," *Ann. Int. Med.* **11**, 801–818 (1937).
68. Dameshek, W., and Ingall, M., "Agranulocytosis (malignant neutropenia). Report of nine cases, two with recovery," *Am. J. M. Sc.* **181**, 502–522 (1931).
69. Dameshek, W., and Miller, E. B., "The megakaryocytes in idiopathic thrombocytopenic purpura, a form of hypersplenism," *Blood* **1**, 27–51 (1946).
70. Dausset, J., "Agranulocytoses et leucopénies immunologiques aspects sérologiques et sérologie des leucocytes en général," *Sang* **25**, 683–706 (1954).
71. Dawbarn, R. Y., Earlam, F., and Evans, W. H., "The relation of the blood platelets to thrombosis after operation and parturition," *J. Path. & Bact.* **31**, 833–873 (1928).

72. Degos, R., Ossipowski, B., and Baranger, H., "Étude Critique des Leucémies à Monocytes," *La Presse Médicale* **70**, 1441–1445 (1954).
73. Diggs, L. W., and Bibb, J., "The erythrocyte in sickle cell anemia; morphology, size, hemoglobin content, fragility and sedimentation rate," *J. A. M. A.* **112**, 695–700 (1939).
74. Diggs, L. W., and Sirridge, M. S., "A study of the sternal marrow and peripheral blood of fifty-five patients with plasma cell myeloma," *J. Lab. & Clin. Med.* **32**, 167–177 (1947).
75. Doan, C. A., Cunningham, R. S., and Sabin, F. R., *Experimental studies on the origin and maturation of avian and mammalian red blood cells*, Carnegie Institution of Washington, Pub. No. 361 (1925), pp. 163–226 (Contributions to embryology).
76. Doan, C. A., and Reinhart, H. L., "The basophil granulocyte, basophilcytosis, and myeloid leukemia, basophil and "mixed granule" types; an experimental, clinical, and pathological study, with the report of a new syndrome," *Am. J. Clin. Path.* **11**, 1–40 (1941).
77. Doan, C. A., and Sabin, F. R., "Normal and pathological fragmentation of red blood cells; the phagocytosis of these fragments by desquamated endothelial cells of the blood stream; the correlation of the peroxidase reaction with phagocytosis in mononuclear cells," *J. Exper. Med.* **43**, 839–850 (1926).
78. Doniach, I., Grüneberg, H., and Pearson, J. E. G., "The occurrence of siderocytes in adult human blood," *J. Path. & Bact.* **55**, 23–31 (1943).
79. Downey, H., "Monocytic leucemia and leucemic reticulo-endotheliosis," in Downey, H., *Handbook of hematology* (Paul B. Hoeber, Inc., New York, Vol. 2, 1938) pp. 1275–1333.
80. Downey, H., "Diseases of the blood," in Bell, E. T., *A textbook of pathology* (Lea & Febiger, Philadelphia, 1934) p. 675.
81. Downey, H., Major, S. G., and Noble, J. F., "Leukemoid blood pictures of the myeloid type," *Folia haemat.* **41**, 493–511 (1930).
82. Downey, H., and McKinlay, C. A., "Acute lymphadenosis compared with acute lymphatic leukemia," *Arch. Int. Med.* **32**, 82–112 (1923).
83. Duke, W. W., "Causes of variation in the platelet count," *Arch. Int. Med.* **11**, 100–120 (1913).
84. Ehrlich, P., "Über schwere anämische Zustände," *Verhandl. d. Kong. f. inn. Med.* **11**, 33–64, 1892.
85. Ehrlich, P., *Farbenanalytische Untersuchungen zur Histologie und Klinik des Blutes* (Hirschwald, Berlin, 1891).
86. Ehrlich, P., and Lazarus, A., *Anaemia* (Rebman Co., New York, Eng. ed., 1910), p. 68.
87. Emerson, C. P., Ham, T. H., and Castle, W. B., "Hemolytic action of certain organic oxidants derived from sulfanilamide, phenylhydrazine and hydroquinone," *J. Clin. Investigation* **20**, 451 (1941).
88. Emmel, V. E., "A study of the erythrocytes in a case of severe anemia with elongated and sickle-shaped red blood corpuscles," *Arch. Int. Med.* **20**, 586–598 (1917).
89. Epstein, R. D., "Cells of the megakaryocyte series in pernicious anemia: in particular the effect of specific therapy," *Am. J. Path.* **25**, 239–251 (1949).
90. Evans, F. A., "Observations on the origin and status of the so-called 'transitional' white blood cell," *Arch. Int. Med.* **17**, 1–12 (1916).
91. Evans, T. S., "Monocytic leukemia (general review of subject)," *Medicine* **21**, 421–456 (1942).
92. Falconer, E. H., "The clinical significance of punctate basophilia in the erythrocyte," *Ann. Int. Med.* **12**, 1429–1441 (1939).
93. Ferrata, A., and Franco, E., "Cellule istiodi (emoistioblasti) e loro derivati nel sangue circolante," *Arch. per le sc. med.* **42**, 109–122 (1919).
94. Ferrata, A., and Storti, E., *Le malattie del sangue manule per medici e studenti*, (Societe Editrice Libraria, Milan, 1946).
95. Fertman, M. H., and Doan, C. A., "Irreversible toxic 'inclusion body' anemia. A rarely recognized syndrome; clinical and experimental studies," *Blood* **3**, 349–360 (1948).
96. Fertman, M. H., and Fertman, M. B., "Toxic anemias and Heinz bodies," *Medicine* **34**, 131–192 (1955).
97. Foord, A. G., Parsons, L., and Butt, E. M., "Leukemic reticulo-endotheliosis (monocytic leukemia) with report of cases," *J. A. M. A.* **101**, 1859–1866 (1933).
98. Foot, N. C., "The endothelial phagocyte. A critical review," *Anat. Rec.* **30**, 15–51 (1925).
99. Forkner, C. E., "Clinical and pathologic differentiation of the acute leukemias; with special reference to acute monocytic leukemia," *Arch. Int. Med.* **53**, 1–34 (1934).
100. Frerichs, J. B., "The influence of a monocytosis of the peripheral blood stream upon the cellular character of an acute inflammation," *Bull. Johns Hopkins Hosp.* **74**, 49–54, 1944.
101. Fuente, V. de la, "Megakaryocytes in normal and in thrombocytopenic individuals," *Blood* **4**, 614–630 (1949).
102. Gall, E. A., "Diagnostic value of supravital staining in infectious mononucleosis," *Am. J. M. Sc.* **194**, 546–554 (1937).
103. Gall, E. A., and Mallory, T. B., "Malignant lymphoma, a clinico-pathologic survey of 618 cases," *Am. J. Path.* **18**, 381–430 (1942).
104. Gardner, F. H., and Mettier, S. R., "Lymphocytic leukemoid reaction of the blood associated with miliary tuberculosis," *Blood* **4**, 767–775 (1949).
105. Giffin, H. Z., and Holloway, J. K., "A review of twenty-eight cases of purpura hemorrhagica in which splenectomy was performed," *Am. J. M. Sc.* **170**, 186–206 (1925).
106. Goldner, F. M., and Mann, W. N., "The statistical error of the differential white count," *Guy's Hosp. Rep.* **88**, 54–65 (1938).

107. Goodwin, A. F., "Some new observations on Auer bodies in acute myelogenous leukemia," *Folia haemat.* **51**, 359–366 (1934).

108. Gordin, R., "Toxic granulation in leukocytes, development and relation to cloudy swelling," *Acta med. Scandinav.* **143**, Supplement 270 (1952).

109. Greenberg, M. S., Kass, E. H., and Castle, W. B., "Studies on the destruction of red blood cells. XII. Factors influencing the role of S hemoglobin in the pathologic physiology of sickle cell anemia and related disorders," *J. Clin. Investigation* **36**, 833–843 (1957).

110. Griggs, R. C., and Harris, J. W., "The biophysics of the variants of sickle-cell disease," *A. M. A. Arch. Int. Med.* **97**, 315–326 (1956).

111. Grüneberg, H., "The anemia of flexed-tailed mice. II. Siderocytes," *J. Genetics* **44**, 246–271 (1942).

112. Grüneberg, H., "Siderocytes: a new kind of erythrocyte," *Nature* **148**, 114–115 (1941).

113. Haden, R. L., "The mechanism of the increased fragility of the erythrocytes in congenital hemolytic jaundice," *Am. J. M. Sc.* **188**, 441–461 (1934).

114. Hahn, E. V., and Gillespie, E. B., "Sickle cell anemia: report of a case greatly improved by splenectomy," *Arch. Int. Med.* **39**, 233–254 (1927).

115. Hall, B. E., and Watkins, C. H., "Myelogenous leukemia changing to monocytic leukemia," *Am. J. Clin. Path.* **11**, 443–459 (1941).

116. Ham, T. H., *A syllabus of laboratory examinations in clinical diagnosis* (Harvard University Press, 1950; rev. L. B. Page and P. J. Culver, 1960).

117. Ham, T. H., Castle, W. B., Gardner, F. H., and Daland, G. A., "Laboratory diagnosis of polycythemia and anemia," *New England J. Med.* **243**, 815–827, 860–872 (1950).

118. Ham, T. H., Shen, S. C., Fleming, E. M., and Castle, W. B., "Studies on the destruction of red blood cells. IV. Thermal injury: Action of heat in causing increased spheroidicity, osmotic and mechanical fragilities and hemolysis of erythrocytes; observations on the mechanisms of destruction of such erythrocytes in dogs and in a patient with a fatal thermal burn," *Blood* **3**, 373–403 (1948).

119. Ham, T. H., Wiseman, R., Jr., and Hinz, C. F., Jr.," "Mechanisms of destruction of red cells in certain hemolytic conditions," *A. M. A. Arch. Int. Med.* **96**, 574–592 (1956).

120. Harris, J. W., Brewster, H. H., Ham, T. H., and Castle, W. B., "Studies on the destruction of red blood cells. X. The biophysics and biology of sickle-cell disease," *A. M. A. Arch. Int. Med.* **97**, 145–168 (1956).

121. Hartz, W. H., Jr., and Schwartz, S. O., "Hemoglobin C disease. Report of 4 cases," *Blood* **10**, 235–246 (1955).

122. Havens, W. P., and Marck, R. E., "The leukocyte response of patients with experimentally induced infectious hepatitis," *Am. J. M. Sc.* **212**, 129–138 (1946).

123. Heath, C. W., and Daland, G. A., "The life of reticulocytes; experiments on their maturation," *Arch. Int. Med.* **46**, 533–551 (1930).

124. Heck, F. J., and Hall, B. E., "Leukemoid reactions of myeloid type," *J. A. M. A.* **112**, 95–101 (1939).

125. Heinz, R., "Morphologische Veränderungen der rothen Blutkörperchen durch Gifte," *Virchows Arch. f. path. Anat.* **122**, 112–116 (1890).

126. Hematology Department, U.S. Naval Medical School, *Hematology* (U.S. Naval Medical School, National Naval Medical Center, Bethesda, Maryland, 1945).

127. Hertz, S., and Lerman, J., "The blood picture in exophthalmic goitre and its changes resulting from iodine and operation — a study by means of the supravital technique," *J. Clin. Investigation* **11**, 1179–1196 (1932).

128. Hickling, R. A., "Chronic non-leukaemic myelosis," *Quart. J. Med.* **6**, 253–275 (1937).

129. Hill, J. M., and Duncan, C. N., "Leukemoid reactions," *Am. J. M. Sc.* **201**, 847–857 (1941).

130. Hill, L. W., "Report on leucocyte inclusion bodies," *Boston M. & S. J.* **170**, 792–794 (1914).

131. Hills, A. G., Forsham, P. H., and Finch, C. A., "Changes in circulating leukocytes induced by the administration of pituitary adrenocorticotropic hormone (ACTH) in man," *Blood* **3**, 755–768 (1948).

132. Holbook, A. A., "The blood picture in chicken pox," *Arch. Int. Med.* **68**, 294–308 (1941).

133. Huët, G. J., "Über eine bisher undekannte familiäre Anomalie de Leukocyten," *Klin. Wchnschr.* **11**, 1264–1266 (1932).

134. Humble, J. G., Anderson, I., White, J. C., and Freeman, T., "A family illustrating the double inheritance of the sickle cell trait and of Mediterranean anaemia," *J. Clin. Path.* **7**, 201–208, 1954.

135. Hunter, F. T., "Drug or protein allergy as a cause of agranulocytosis and certain types of purpura," *New England J. Med.* **213**, 663–674 (1935).

136. Isaacs, R., "The refractive granule red blood corpuscle; its behavior and significance," *Anat. Rec.* **29**, 299–313 (1925).

137. Isaacs, R., Brock, B., and Minot, G. R., "The resistance of immature erythrocytes to heat," *J. Clin. Investigation* **1**, 425–433 (1925).

138. Israels, M. C. G., "The reticuloses, a clinicopathological study," *Lancet* **2**, 525–530 (1953).

139. Israels, M. C. G., *An atlas of bone-marrow pathology* (Grune & Stratton, New York, 1948).

140. Itano, H. A., "Clinical states associated with alterations of the hemoglobin molecule," *A. M. A. Arch Int. Med.* **96**, 287–297 (1955).

141. Itano, H. A., and Pauling, L., "A rapid diagnostic test for sickle cell anemia," *Blood* **4**, 66–68 (1949).

142. Jackson, H., Jr., "The protean character of the leukemias and of the leukemoid states," *New England J. Med.* **220**, 175–181 (1939).

143. Jackson, H., Jr., and Merrill, D., "Agranulocytosis

angina associated with the menstrual cycle," *New England J. Med.* **210**, 175–176 (1934).

144. Jackson, H., Jr., and Parker, F., Jr., "Agranulocytosis: its etiology and treatment," *New England J. Med.* **212**, 137–148 (1935).

145. Jackson, H., Jr., and Parker, F., Jr., *Hodgkin's disease and allied disorders* (Oxford University Press, New York, 1947).

146. Jackson, H., Jr., Parker, F., Jr., and Bethea, J. M., "Studies of diseases of the lymphoid and myeloid tissues. II. Plasmatocytoma and their relation to multiple myelomata," *Am. J. M. Sc.* **181**, 169–180 (1931).

147. Jackson, H., Jr., Parker, F., Jr., and Lemon, H. M., "Agnogenic myeloid metaplasia of the spleen; a syndrome simulating other more definite hematologic disorders," *New England J. Med.* **222**, 985–994 (1940).

148. Jaffee, R. H., "Aleukemic myelosis," *Arch. Path. & Lab. Med.* **3**, 56–72 (1927).

149. Jarcho, S., "Diffusely infiltrative carcinoma, a hitherto undescribed correlation of several varieties of tumor metastasis," *Arch. Path.* **22**, 674–696 (1936).

150. Jones, O., in H. Downey, ed., *Handbook of hematology* (Hoeber, New York, 1938) p. 2101.

151. Jordan, W. S., Prouty, R. L., Heinle, R. W., and Dingle, J. H., "The mechanism of hemolysis in paroxysmal cold hemoglobinuria," *Blood* **7**, 387–403 (1942).

152. Jordans, G. H. W., "Hereditary granulation anomaly of the leucocytes (Alder)," *Acta med. Scandinav.* **129**, 348–351 (1948).

153. Kaplan, E., Zuelzer, W. W., and Neel, J. V., "A new inherited abnormality of hemoglobin and its interaction with sickle cell hemoglobin," *Blood* **6**, 1240–1259 (1951).

154. Kaplan, E., Zuelzer, W. W., and Neel, J. V., "Further studies on hemoglobin C; II. The hematologic effects of hemoglobin C alone and in combination with sickle cell hemoglobin," *Blood* **8**, 735–746 (1953).

155. Kennedy, P. C., and Finland, M., "Fatal agranulocytosis from sulfathiazole," *J. A. M. A.* **116**, 295–296 (1941).

156. Kleeman, C. R., "Lymphocytic leukemoid reaction associated with primary carcinoma of the breast," *Am. J. Med.* **10**, 522–527 (1951).

157. Klein, A., Hussar, A. E., and Bornstein, S., "Pelger-Huët anomaly of the leukocytes," *New England J. Med.* **253**, 1057–1062 (1955).

158. Kolouch, F., Good, R. A., and Campbell, B., "The reticulo-endothelial origin of the bone marrow plasma cells in hypersensitive states," *J. Lab. & Clin. Med.* **32**, 749–755 (1947).

159. Korst, D. R., Clatanoff, D. V., and Schilling, R. F., "On myelofibrosis," *A. M. A. Arch. Int. Med.* **97**, 169–183 (1956).

160. Krumbhaar, E. B., "Leukemoid blood pictures in various clinical conditions," *Am. J. M. Sc.* **172**, 519–533 (1926).

161. Krumbhaar, E. B., "The changes produced in the blood picture by removal of the normal mammalian spleen," *Am. J. M. Sc.* **184**, 215–228 (1932).

162. Kugel, M. A., and Rosenthal, N., "Pathological changes in polymorphonuclear leukocytes during progress of infections," *Am. J. M. Sc.* **183**, 657–667 (1932).

163. Kunkel, H. G., and Wallenius, G., "New hemoglobin in normal adult blood," *Science* **122**, 288 (1955).

164. Lawrence, J. S., "Leukopenia: its classification, etiology and treatment," *Tr. and Stud., Coll. Physicians, Philadelphia* **14**, 1–14 (1946).

165. Lawrence, J. S., Neel, J. V., and Itano, H., "Hemolytic anemia presumably due to coexistence of the gene for thalassemia and sickling," *Tr. A. Am. Physicians* **65**, 203–213 (1952).

166. Lawrence, J. S., and Todd, H., "Variations in the characteristics of lymphocytes in supravital preparations," *Folia haemat.* **44**, 318–331 (1931).

167. Lee, R. I., and Minot, G. R., "The significance of blood platelets," *Cleveland M. J.* **16**, 65–88 (1917).

168. Lee, R. I., Vincent, B., and Robertson, O. H., "Immediate results of splenectomy in pernicious anemia," *J. A. M. A.* **65**, 216–220 (1915).

169. Lehman, H., "Variations of haemoglobin synthesis in man," *Acta Genetica et Statistica Medica* **6**, 413–429 (1956–1957).

170. Leitner, S. J., *Bone marrow biopsy: Haemotology in the light of sternal puncture* (trans. and rev. by C. J. C. Britton and E. Neumark; Grune and Stratton, New York, 1949).

171. Lesses, M. F., and Gargill, S. L., "Thiouracil as a cause of neutropenia and agranulocytosis," *New England J. Med.* **233**, 803–811 (1945).

172. Lichtenstein, L., "Histiocytosis X: Integration of eosinophilic granuloma of bone, 'Letterer-Siwe Disease' and Schüller-Christian disease as related manifestations of a single nosologic entity," *A. M. A. Arch. Path.* **56**, 84–102 (1953).

173. Lie-Injo, Luan Eng, "Haemoglobin E in Indonesia," *Nature* **176**, 469–470 (1955).

174. Lie-Injo, Luan Eng, and Jo Kian Tjoy, "Cooley's anaemia in children in Indonesia," *Docum. de med. geogr. et trop.* **7**, 30–42 (1955).

175. Lie-Injo, Luan Eng, Poey Seng Hin, Kho Lien Keng, and Endenburg, P. M., "Chronic hypochromic microcytic anaemia associated with haemoglobin H," *Acta haemat.* **18**, 156–167 (1957).

176. Lipton, E. L., "Elliptocytosis with hemolytic anemia; the effect of splenectomy," *Pediat.* **15**, 67–83 (1955).

177. Lucey, H. C., "Fortuitous factors affecting the leucocyte count in blood from the ear," *J. Clin. Path.* **3**, 146–151 (1950).

178. MacBryde, C. M., and Charles, C. M., "Differential diagnosis of rubella; use of the Schilling leuko-

cyte count," *Arch. Int. Med.* **56**, 935–943 (1935).

179. McFadzean, A. J. S., and Davis, L. J., "Iron staining erythrocytic inclusions with special reference to acquired haemolytic anaemia," *Glasgow M. J.* **28**, 237–279 (1947).
180. Mackay, W., "The blood-platelet: its clinical significance," *Quart. J. Med.* **24**, 285–328 (1931).
181. Madison, F. W., and Squier, T. L., "The etiology of primary granulocytopenia (agranulocytic angina)," *J. A. M. A.* **102**, 755–759 (1934).
182. Mainland, D., Coady, B. K., and Joseph, S., "Observational variation in the differential count," *Folia haemat.* **54**, 8–21 (1936).
183. March, H. W., Schlyen, S. M., and Schwartz, S. E., "Mediterranean hemopathic syndromes (Cooley's anemia) in adults," *Am. J. Med.* **13**, 46–57 (1952).
184. Marchal, G., and Bargeton, A., "Difficultés de diagnostic entre Maladie de Hodgkin et leucémie à monocytes," *Sang* **7**, 321–327 (1933).
185. Maximow, A. A., and Bloom, W., *A textbook of histology* (W. B. Saunders, Philadelphia, ed. 5, 1948) p. 89.
186. McIntosh, R., and Wood, C. L., "An inquiry into the genetic factor in Cooley's anemia," *Am. J. Dis. Child.* **64**, 192–194 (1942).
187. Medlar, E. M., "An evaluation of the leucocytic reaction in the blood as found in cases of tuberculosis," *Am. Rev. Tuberc.* **20**, 312–346 (1929).
188. Menkin, V., "Relative lymphocytosis in hyperthyroidism," *Arch. Int. Med.* **42**, 419–424 (1928).
189. Merrill, D., and Jackson, H., Jr., "Renal complications of leukemia," *New England J. Med.* **228**, 271–276 (1943).
190. Michels, N. A., "The plasma cell," *Arch. Path.* **11**, 775–793 (1931).
191. Mickler, E. E., and Diggs, L. W., "The detection of the sickle cell trait; a comparison of the sealed moist preparation using capillary blood collected during venous stasis and the sodium bisulfite method," *Am. J. Clin. Path.* **20**, 861–864 (1950).
192. Minnich, V., Na-Nakorn, S., Chongchareonsuk, S., and Kochaseni, S., "Mediterranean anemia. A study of thirty-two cases in Thailand," *Blood* **9**, 1–23 (1954).
193. Minot, G. R., "Megacaryocytes in the peripheral circulation," *J. Exper. Med.* **35**, 1–7 (1922).
194. Minot, G. R., and Buckman, T. E., "Erythremia (Polycythemia rubra vera). The development of anemia; the relation to leukemia; consideration of the basal metabolism, blood formation and destruction and fragility of the red cells," *Am. J. M. Sc.* **166**, 469–489 (1923).
195. Minot, G. R., and Buckman, T. E., "The blood platelets in the leukemias," *Am. J. M. Sc.* **169**, 477–485 (1925).
196. Minot, G. R., and Jones, C. M., "Infectious (catarrhal) jaundice. An attempt to establish a clinical entity," *Boston M. & S. J.* **189**, 531–551 (1923).
197. Minot, G. R., and Smith, L. W., "The blood in tetrachlorethane poisoning," *Arch. Int. Med.* **28**, 687–702 (1921).
198. Moeschlin, S., "Immunological agranulocytosis (clinical aspects)," *Sang* **25**, 679–682 (1954).
199. Monasterio, G., and Gigli, G., "Histioleukaemias and acute leukaemias," *Acta med. Scandinav.* **140**, 381–394 (1951).
200. Montgomery, H., and Watkins, C. H., "Monocytic leukemia. Cutaneous manifestations of the Naegeli and Schilling types; hematologic differentiation," *A. M. A. Arch. Int. Med.* **60**, 51–63 (1937).
201. Morissette, L., and Watkins, C. H., "Multiple myeloma, diagnostic value of the blood smear," *Proc. Staff Meet., Mayo Clin.* **17**, 433–439 (1942).
202. Morris, R. S., "Nuclear particles in the erythrocytes," *Arch. Int. Med.* **3**, 93–97 (1909).
203. Moss, W. T., and Ackerman, L. V., "Plasma cell leukemia," *Blood* **1**, 396–406 (1946).
204. Motulsky, A. G., "Genetic and haematological significance of hemoglobin H," *Nature* **178**, 1055–1056 (1956).
205. Motulsky, A. G., Luttgens, W. F., Patterson, W., and Rotter, R., "Splenic infarction precipitated by airplane flight in patients with sicklemia," *Clin. Research Proc.* **3**, 51 (1955).
206. Mugrage, E. R., and Andresen, M. I., "Value for red blood cells of average infants and children," *Am. J. Dis. Child.* **51**, 775–791 (1936).
207. Naegeli, O., *Blutkrankheiten und Blutdiagnostik* (J. Springer, Berlin, (1931).
208. Na-Nakorn, S., and Minnich, V., "Studies on hemoglobin E. III. Homozygous hemoglobin E and variants of thalassemia and hemoglobin E. A family study," *Blood* **12**, 529–538 (1957).
209. Neel, J. V., "The inheritance of sickle cell anemia," *Science* **110**, 64–66 (1949).
210. Neel, J. V., "The inheritance of the sickling phenomenon with particular reference to sickle cell disease," *Blood* **6**, 389–412 (1951).
211. Neel, J. V., "Abnormal forms of hemoglobin from a genetic point of view," *A. M. A. Arch. Int. Med.* **96**, 555–558 (1956).
212. Neel, J. V., "The genetics of human haemoglobin differences; problems and perspectives," *Ann. Human Genet.* **21**, 1–30 (1956).
213. Neel, J. V., "Human hemoglobin types; their epidemiologic implications," *New England J. Med.* **256**, 161–171 (1957).
214. Neel, J. V., Itano, H. A., and Lawrence, J. S., "Two cases of sickle cell disease presumably due to the combination of the genes for thalassemia and sickle cell hemoglobin," *Blood* **8**, 434–443 (1953).
215. Neel, J. V., Kaplan, E., and Zuelzer, W. W., "Further studies on hemoglobin C. I. A description of three additional families segregating for hemoglobin C and sickle cell hemoglobin," *Blood* **8**, 724–734 (1953).
216. Neel, J. V., and Valentine, W. N., "The frequency of thalassemia," *Am. J. M. Sc.* **209**, 568–572 (1945).

217. Olef, I., "The differential platelet count; its clinical significance," *Arch. Int. Med.* **57**, 1163–1185 (1936).
218. Orchard, N. P., "Letterer-Siwe's syndrome; report of a case with unusual peripheral blood changes," *Arch. Dis. Childhood* **25**, 151–155 (1950).
219. Osgood, E. E., "Monocytic leukemia, report of 6 cases and review of 127 cases," *Arch. Int. Med.* **59**, 931–951 (1937).
220. Osgood, E. E., Baker, R. L., Brownlee, B. A., Osgood, M. W., Ellis, D. M., and Cohen, W., "Total, differential and absolute leukocyte counts and sedimentation rates of healthy children four to seven years of age," *A. M. A. Am. J. Dis. Child.* **58**, 61–70 (1939).
221. Ottander, O., "Hochgradige Endotheliose im Blut bei Endocarditis lenta," *Acta med. Scandinav.* **63**, 336–354 (1925–1926).
222. Owren, P. A., "Cyclic agranulocytosis," *Acta med. Scandinav.* **134**, 87–97 (1949).
223. Owren, P. A., "Congenital hemolytic jaundice. The pathogenesis of the hemolytic crisis," *Blood* **3**, 231–248 (1948).
224. Pappenheim, A., *Clinical examination of the blood and its technique. A manual for students and practitioners* (trans. and adapt. from German by R. Donaldson; Wood, New York, 1914).
225. Pappenheimer, A. M., Thompson, W. P., Parker, D. D., and Smith, K. E., "Anaemia associated with unidentified erythrocyte inclusions after splenectomy," *Quart. J. Med.* **14**, 75–100 (1945).
226. Parsons, W. B., Cooper T., and Scheifly, C. H., "Anemia in bacterial endocarditis," *J. A. M. A.* **153**, 14–16 (1953).
227. Patek, A. J., Jr., and Castle, W. B., "Plasma cell leukemia," *Am. J. M. Sc.* **191**, 788–794 (1936).
228. Paul, J. R., and Bunnell, W. W., "The presence of heterophile antibodies in infectious mononucleosis," *Am. J. M. Sc.* **183**, 90–104 (1932).
229. Pauling, L., Itano, H. A., Singer, S. J., and Wells, I. C., "Sickle cell anemia, a molecular disease," *Science* **110**, 543–548 (1949).
230. Pearse, A. G. E., "Nature of Russell bodies and Kurloff bodies, observations on cytochemistry of plasma cells and reticulum cells," *J. Clin. Path.* **2**, 81–90 (1949).
231. Pepper, O. H. P., "The hematology of subacute streptococcus viridans endocarditis," *J. A. M. A.* **89**, 1377–1380 (1927).
232. Pohle, F. J., "The blood platelet count in relation to the menstrual cycle in normal women," *Am. J. M. Sc.* **197**, 40–47 (1939).
233. Powell, W. N., Rodarte, J. G., and Neel, J. V., "The occurrence in a family of Sicilian ancestry of the traits for both sickling and thalassemia," *Blood* **5**, 887–897 (1950).
234. Price-Jones, C., *Red blood cell diameters* (Oxford Medical Publications, London, 1933).
235. Ranney, H. M., "Observations on the inheritance of sickle-cell hemoglobin and hemoglobin C," *J. Clin. Investigation* **33**, 1634–1641 (1954).
236. Rawson, R., Parker, F., Jr., and Jackson, H., Jr., "Industrial solvents as possible etiologic agents in myeloid metaplasia," *Science* **93**, 541 (1941).
237. Rebuck, J. W., "The structure of the giant cells in the blood-forming organs," *J. Lab. & Clin. Med.* **32**, 660–699 (1947).
238. Reich, C., "A case of adenocarcinoma of the sigmoid with lymphatic leukemia blood picture," *Am. J. Cancer* **26**, 781–782 (1936).
239. Reich, C., and Rumsey, W., Jr., "Agnogenic myeloid metaplasia of the spleen; report of five cases illustrating diagnostic difficulties and danger of splenectomy and radiation therapy," *J. A. M. A.* **118**, 1200–1204 (1942).
240. Reiman, H. A., "The blood platelets in pneumococcus infections," *J. Exper. Med.* **40**, 553–565 (1924).
241. Reschad, H., and Schilling-Torgau, V., "Ueber eine neue Leukämie durch echte Uebergangsformen (Splenozyten leukämie) und ihre Bedeutung für die Selbstandigkeit dieser Zellen," *München. med. Wchnschr.* **60**, 1981–1989 (1913).
242. Reznikoff, P., "White blood cell counts in convalescence from infectious diseases," *Am. J. M. Sc.* **184**, 167–184 (1932).
243. Rich, A., "Studies on the hemoglobin of Cooley's anemia and Cooley's trait," *Proc. Nat. Acad. Sc.* **38**, 187–196 (1952).
244. Richter, M. N., "The presence of Auer bodies in leukemic tissues," *Arch. Int. Med.* **31**, 677–685 (1923).
245. Richter, M. N., "Observations on the hemohistioblast of Ferrata," *Am. J. M. Sc.* **169**, 336–445 (1925).
246. Rigas, D. A., Koler, R. D., and Osgood, E. E., "New hemoglobin possessing higher electrophoretic mobility than normal adult hemoglobin," *Science* **121**, 372 (1955).
247. Rolland, C. F., and Davidson, L. S. P., "A case of cyclic neutropenia," *Edinburgh M. J.* **57**, 205–210 (1950).
248. Rous, P., and Robertson, O. H., "The normal fate of erythrocytes. I. The findings in healthy animals," *J. Exper. Med.* **25**, 651–663 (1917).
249. Rowley, M. W., "The occurrence of atypical phagocytic cells in the circulating blood," *New York M. J.* **85**, 674–675 (1907).
250. Rowley, M. W., "A fatal anaemia with enormous numbers of circulating phagocytes," *J. Exper. Med.* **10**, 78–96 (1908).
251. Sabin, F. R., and Doan, C. A., "The presence of desquamated endothelial cells, the so-called clasmatocytes, in normal mammalian blood," *J. Exper. Med.* **43**, 823–837 (1926).
252. Sabin, F. R., Doan, C. A., and Cunningham, R. S., "Discrimination of two types of phagocytic cells in the connective tissues by the supravital tech-

nique," *Carnegie Institution of Washington Pub. No.* **361** (1925) p. 125 (Contributions to embryology, No. 82).

253. Sandoz, *Atlas of haematology* (Sandoz, Ltd., Basle, Switzerland and Sandoz Pharmaceuticals, New York, 1952).
254. Schilling, T. V., "Ein praktisch und zur Demontration brachbarer Differential leukozytometer mit Arnethscher Verschiebung des Blutbildes," *Deutsch med. Wchnschr.* **37**, 1159–1163 (1911).
255. Schleicher, E. M., "The origin and nature of the Cabot-ring bodies of erythrocytes," *J. Lab. & Clin. Med.* **27**, 983–1000 (1942).
256. Schneider, R. G., "Incidence of hemoglobin C trait in 505 normal negroes; a family with homozygous hemoglobin C and sickle cell trait union," *J. Lab. & Clin. Med.* **44**, 133–144 (1954).
257. Schwartz, S. O., and Motto, S. A., "The diagnostic significance of "burr" red blood cells," *Am. J. M. Sc.* **218**, 563–566 (1949).
258. Schwartz, H. C., Spaet, T. H., Zuelzer, W. W., Neel, J. V., Robinson, A. R., and Kaufman, S. F., "Combinations of hemoglobin G, hemoglobin S and thalassemia occurring in one family," *Blood* **12**, 238–250 (1957).
259. Shen, S. C., Fleming, E. M., and Castle, W. B., "Studies on the destruction of red blood cells. V. Irreversibly sickled erythrocytes: their experimental production in vitro," *Blood* **4**, 498–504 (1949).
260. Shen, S. C., Ham, T. H., and Fleming, E. M., "Studies on the destruction of red blood cells. III. Mechanism and complications of hemoglobinuria in patients with thermal burns, spherocytosis and increased osmotic fragility of erythrocytes," *New England J. Med.* **229**, 701–713 (1943).
261. Silvestroni, E., and Bianco, I., "Genetic aspects of sickle cell anemia and microdrepanocytic disease," *Blood* **7**, 429–435 (1952).
262. Singer, K., "Hereditary hemolytic disorders associated with abnormal hemoglobins," *Am. J. Med.* **18**, 633–652 (1955).
263. Singer, K., Chapman, A. Z., Goldberg, S. R., Rubinstein, H. M., and Rosenblum, S. A., "Studies on abnormal hemoglobins. IX. Pure (homozygous) hemoglobin C disease," *Blood* **9**, 1023–1031 (1954).
264. Singer, K., Chernoff, A. I., and Singer, L., "Studies on abnormal hemoglobins. I. Their demonstration in sickle cell anemia and other hematologic disorders by means of alkali denaturation," *Blood* **6**, 413–435 (1951).
265. Singer, K., Fisher, B., and Perlstein, M. A., "Acanthrocytosis, a genetic erythrocytic malformation," *Blood* **7**, 577–591 (1952).
266. Singer, K., Josephson, A. M., Singer, L., Heller, P., and Zimmerman, H. J., "Studies on abnormal hemoglobin. XIII. Hemoglobin S — thalassemia disease and hemoglobin C — thalassemia disease in siblings," *Blood* **12**, 593–602 (1957).
267. Singer, K., Kraus, A. P., Singer, L., Rubinstein, H. M., and Goldberg, S. R., "Studies on abnormal hemoglobins. X. A new syndrome: hemoglobin C — thalassemia disease," *Blood* **9**, 1032–1046 (1954).
268. Singer, K., Miller, E. B., and Dameshek, W., "Hematologic changes following splenectomy in man, with particular reference to target cells, hemolytic index and lysolecithin," *Am. J. M. Sc.* **202**, 171–187 (1941).
269. Singer, K., Singer, L., and Goldberg, S. R., "Studies on abnormal hemoglobins. XI. Sickle cell — thalassemia disease in the Negro, the significance of the S + A + F and S + A patterns obtained by hemoglobin analysis," *Blood* **10**, 405–415 (1955).
270. Smith, C. H., "Acute infectious lymphocytosis: a specific infection, report of four cases showing its communicability," *J. A. M. A.* **125**, 342–349 (1944).
271. Smith, E. W., and Conley, C. L., "Filter paper electrophoresis of human hemoglobins with special reference to the incidence and clinical significance of hemoglobin C," *Bull. Johns Hopkins Hosp.* **93**, 94–106 (1953).
272. Smith, E. W., and Conley, C. L., "Clinical features of the genetic variants of sickle cell disease," *Bull. Johns Hopkins Hosp.* **94**, 289–318 (1954).
273. Smith, E. W., and Conley, C. L., "Sicklemia and infarction of the spleen during aerial flight," *Bull. Johns Hopkins Hosp.* **96**, 35–41 (1955).
274. Snell, F. M., Neel, J. V., and Ishibashi, K., "Hematologic studies in Hiroshima and a control city two years after the atomic bombing," *Arch. Int. Med.* **84**, 569–604 (1949).
275. Spence, H. M., and Roberts, G. M., "Extreme leukocytosis and acute hemolytic anemia associated with the administration of sulfanilamide," *New England J. Med.* **222**, 874–876 (1940).
276. "Statement concerning a system of nomenclature for the varieties of human hemoglobin," *Blood* **8**, 386 (1953).
277. Stetson, R. P., "Normal variations in white blood cells under conditions of minimal metabolism," *Arch. Int. Med.* **40**, 488–495 (1927).
278. Stewart, S. G., "Familial eosinophilia," *Am. J. M. Sc.* **185**, 21–29 (1933).
279. Strauss, M. B., and Daland, G. A., "Hereditary ovalocytosis (human eliptical erythrocytes). Observations on ten cases in one family," *New England J. Med.* **217**, 100–103 (1937).
280. Strumia, M. M., *Hematological tables with brief notes* (Bryn Mawr Hospital, Bryn Mawr, Pa., 1937).
281. Sturgeon, P., Itano, H. A., and Bergren, W. R., "Clinical manifestations of inherited abnormal hemoglobins. I. The interaction of hemoglobin S with hemoglobin D," *Blood* **10**, 389–396 (1955).
282. Sturgeon, P., Itano, H. A., and Bergren, W. R., "Clinical manifestations of inherited abnormal hemoglobins, II. Interaction of hemoglobin E and thalassemia trait," *Blood* **10**, 396–404 (1955).
283. Taliaferro, W. H., and Klüver, C., "The hematology

of malaria (plasmodium brasilianum) in Panamanian monkeys; morphology of leucocytes and origin of monocytes and macrophages," *J. Infect. Dis.* **67**, 162–176 (1940).

284. Terry, D. W., Motulsky, A. G., and Rath, C. E., "Homozygous hemoglobin C, a new hereditary hemolytic disease," *New England J. Med.* **251**, 365–373 (1954).

285. Thannhauser, S. J., Lipoidoses, *Diseases of the cellular lipid metabolism* (Oxford Medicine, Ed. Christian, H. A.; Oxford University Press, Inc., New York, 1949).

286. Thewlis, E., and Middleton, W. S., "The leukocytic picture in catarrhal jaundice (cholangitis)," *Am. J. M. Sc.* **169**, 59–68 (1925).

287. Thompson, W. P., "Abnormalities in the white blood cell response (leukemoid, atypical leukemia and leukopenic blood picture)," *Am. J. M. Sc.*, **182**, 334–352 (1931).

288. Thompson, W. P., and Illyne, C. A., "Clinical and hematologic picture resulting from bone marrow replacement," *M. Clin. North America* **24**, 841–853 (1940).

289. Thorn, G. W., Forsham, P. H., Prunty, F. T. G., and Hills, A. G., "The response to pituitary adrenocorticotropic hormone as a test for adrenal cortical insufficiency," *J. A. M. A.* **137**, 1005–1009 (1948).

290. Tileston, W., "Familial shift to the left of the leukocytes (Pelger's nuclear anomaly of the leukocytes) with a report of a case," *Ann. Int. Med.* **11**, 675–681 (1937).

291. Tocantins, L. M., "The mammalian blood platelet in health and disease," *Medicine* **17**, 155–260 (1938).

292. Valentine, W. N., and Neel, J. V., "Hematologic and genetic study of the transmission of thalassemia (Cooley's anemia, Mediterranean anemia)," *Arch. Int. Med.* **74**, 185–196 (1944).

293. Valentine, W. N., and Neel, J. V., "The artificial production and significance of target cells, with special reference to their occurrence in thalassemia (Cooley's erythroblastic anemia)," *Am. J. M. Sc.* **209**, 741–752 (1945).

294. Vaughan, J., and Harrison, C. V., "Leucoerythroblastic anemia and myelosclerosis," *J. Path. & Bact.* **48**, 339–352 (1939).

295. Volini, I. F., Greenspan, I., Ehrlich, L., Gonner, J. A., Felsenfeld, O., and Schwartz, S. O., "Hematopoietic changes during administration of chloramphenicol (chloromycetin)," *J. A. M. A.* **142**, 1333–1335 (1950).

296. Watkins, C. H., and Hall, B. E., "Monocytic leukemia of the Naegeli and Schilling types," *Am. J. Clin. Path.* **10**, 387–396 (1940).

297. Watson, C. J., "The porphyrins and diseases of the blood," in *A symposium on the blood and blood-forming organs* (University of Wisconsin Press, Madison, Wis., 1939), p. 14.

298. Webster, S. H., "Heinz body phenomenon in erythrocytes," *Blood* **4**, 479–497 (1949).

299. Webster, S. H., Liljegren, E. J., and Zimmer, D. J., "Heinz body formation by certain chemical agents," *J. Pharmacol. & Exper. Therap.* **95**, 201–211 (1949).

300. Whipple, G. H., and Bradford, W. L., "Mediterranean disease — thalassemia (erythroblastic anemia of Cooley)," *J. Pediat.* **9**, 279–313 (1936).

301. Whitby, L., and Britton, C. J. C., *Disorders of the blood. Diagnosis, pathology, treatment, technique* (Churchill, London, ed. 6, 1950).

302. White, J. C., and Beavan, G. H., "A review of the varieties of human haemoglobin in health and disease," *J. Clin. Path.* **7**, 175–200 (1954).

303. Wiener, H. A., and Morkovin, D., "Circulating blood eosinophils in acute infectious disease and the eosinopenic response," *Am. J. Med.* **13**, 58–72 (1952).

304. Wilson, C. P., and Cunningham, R. S., "A consideration of the supravital method of studying blood in cases of mononuclear cell response," *Folia haemat.* **38**, 14–29 (1929).

305. Wintrobe, M. M., "The size and hemoglobin content of the erythrocyte," *J. Lab. & Clin. Med.* **17**, 899–912 (1932).

306. Wintrobe, M. M., *Clinical hematology* (Lea & Febiger, Philadelphia, ed. 4, 1956).

307. Wintrobe, M. M., Matthews, E., Pollock, R., and Dobyns, B. M., "A familial hemopoietic disorder in Italian adolescents and adults resembling Mediterranean disease (thalassemia)," *J. A. M. A.* **114**, 1530–1538 (1940).

308. Wiseman, B. K., "Criteria of the age of lymphocytes in the peripheral blood," *J. Exper. Med.* **54**, 271–294 (1931).

309. Wiseman, B. K., and Doan, C. A., "Primary splenic neutropenia; a newly recognized syndrome, closely related to congenital hemolytic icterus and essential thrombocytopenic purpura," *Ann. Int. Med.* **16**, 1097–1117 (1942).

310. Wislocki, G. B., Bunting, H., and Dempsey, E. W., "Further observations on the chemical cytology of megakaryocytes and other cells of hemopoietic tissue." *Anat. Rec.* **98**, 527–537 (1947).

311. Wright, J. H., "The origin and nature of the blood plates," *Boston M. & S. J.* **154**, 643–645 (1906).

312. Wright, J. H., "The histogenesis of the blood platelets," *J. Morphol.* **21**, 263–278 (1910).

313. Wyandt, H., Bancroft, P. M., and Winship, T. O., "Elliptic erythrocytes in man," *Arch. Int. Med.* **68**, 1043–1065 (1941).

314. Zinkham, W. H., and Diamond, L. K., "In vitro erythrophagocytosis in acquired hemolytic anemia," *Blood* **7**, 592–601 (1952).

315. Zuelzer, W. W., and Kaplan, E., "Thalassemia — hemoglobin C disease, a new syndrome presumably due to a combination of genes for the thalassemia and hemoglobin C," *Blood* **9**, 1047–1054 (1954).

316. Zuelzer, W. W., Neel, J. V., and Robinson, A. R., "Abnormal hemoglobins," in *Progress in hematology*, ed. Tocantins, L. M. (Grune and Stratton, New York, 1956), pp. 91–137.

INDEX

PLATES

Plate I. Typical Cells of the Red-Cell Series

(Text on page 8)

Key:

1. Normal red cell
2. Polychromatophilic cell
3. Normoblast

3*a*. Normoblast — pathologic [a]
3*b*. Normoblast with reticulum [b]
3*c*. Normoblast with stippling
3*d*. Normoblast with Howell-Jolly bodies
3*e*. Normoblast with double nucleus
4. Late erythroblast
4*a*. Late erythroblast — pathologic [a]
5. Early erythroblast
5*a*. Early erythroblast — pathologic [a]
6. Proerythroblast
6*a*. Proerythroblast — pathologic [a]
7*a*. Early reticulocyte [b]
7*b*. Intermediate reticulocyte [b]
7*c*. Late reticulocyte [b]
8. Stippled cell
9. Howell-Jolly bodies
10. Siderocytes
10*a*. Siderocyte stained for iron [c]
11. Refractive granule
12. Heinz bodies [d]
13. Nucleated red cells showing mitosis
14. Cabot ring forms
15. Round macrocyte
16. Oval macrocyte
17. Oval cell
18. Pencil form
19. Spheroidal red cell
20. Lunar forms (partially hemolyzed)
21. Crenated cell
22. Burr cell
23. Acanthrocyte
24. Sickled forms
25. Pear-shaped or tailed forms
26. Target cell
27. Irregular forms

[a] These pathologic or abnormal cells are called megaloblasts by many authors.

[b] Vitally stained with brilliant cresyl blue before being counterstained with Wright's stain.

[c] Stained with a solution of equal parts 1 percent hydrochloric acid and 2 percent potassium ferrocyanide and counterstained.

[d] Vitally stained with saturated solution of methyl violet in 0.73 percent sodium chloride.

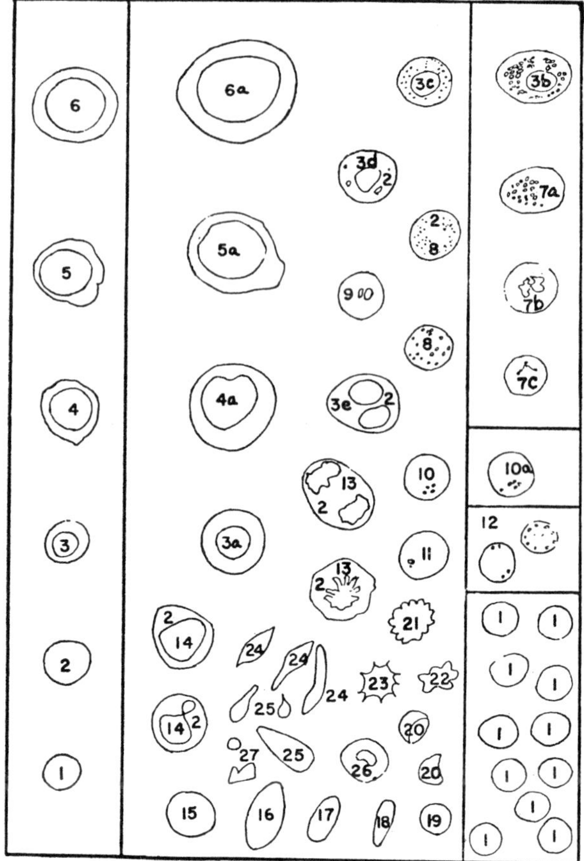

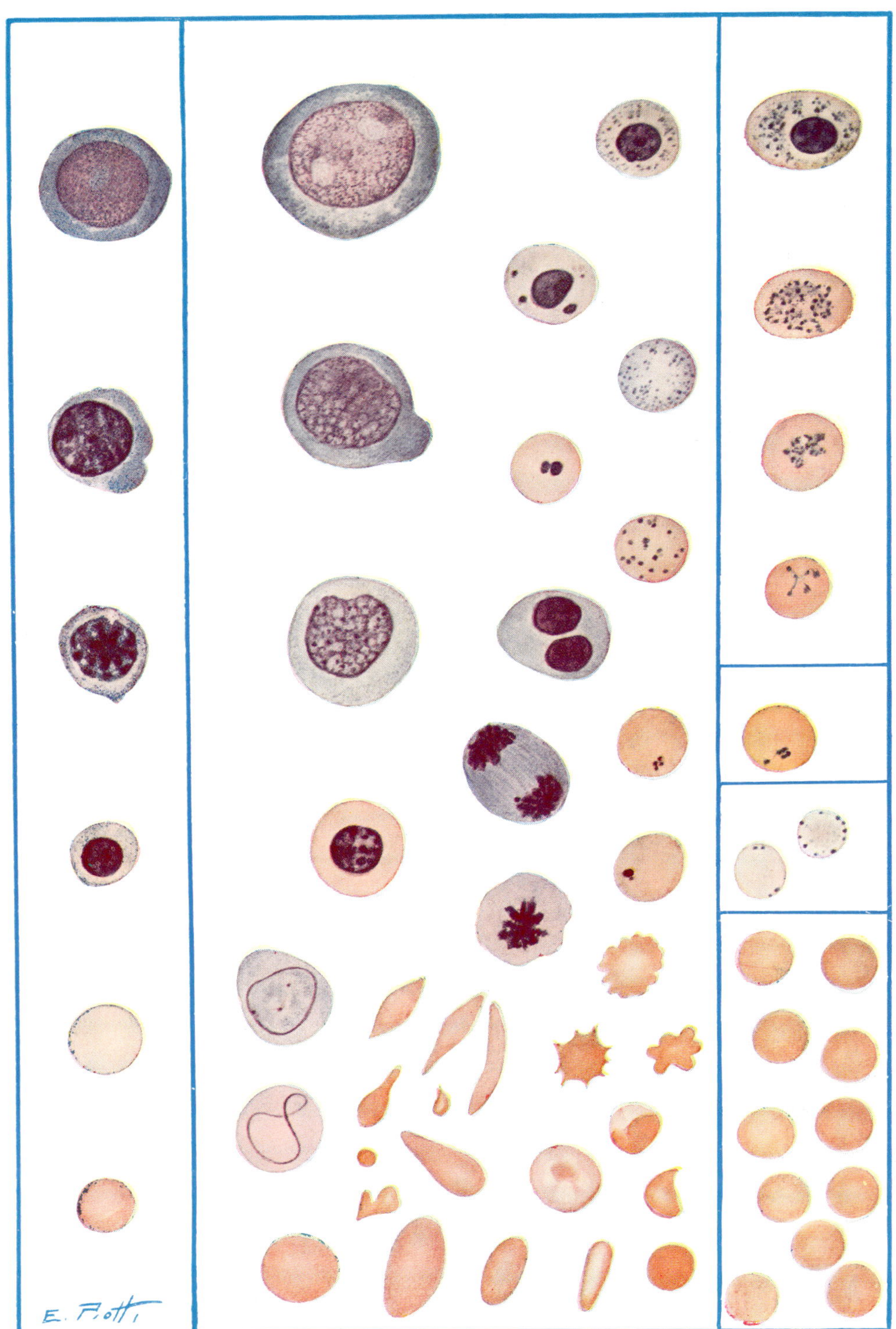

PLATE I. TYPICAL CELLS OF THE RED-CELL SERIES

PLATE II. TYPICAL CELLS OF NORMAL HUMAN BLOOD
(*Text on page 16*)

Key:
1. Normal red cells
2. Platelets
3. Neutrophil, adult
3*a*. Neutrophil, adult (two lobes)
3*b*. Neutrophil, adult, hypersegmented
4. Neutrophil, band form
5*a*. Eosinophil, two lobes
5*b*. Eosinophil, band form
6*a*. Basophil, band form
6*b*. Metamyelocyte, basophilic
7. Lymphocyte, small
8. Lymphocyte, large
9. Monocyte, mature
10. Monocyte, young

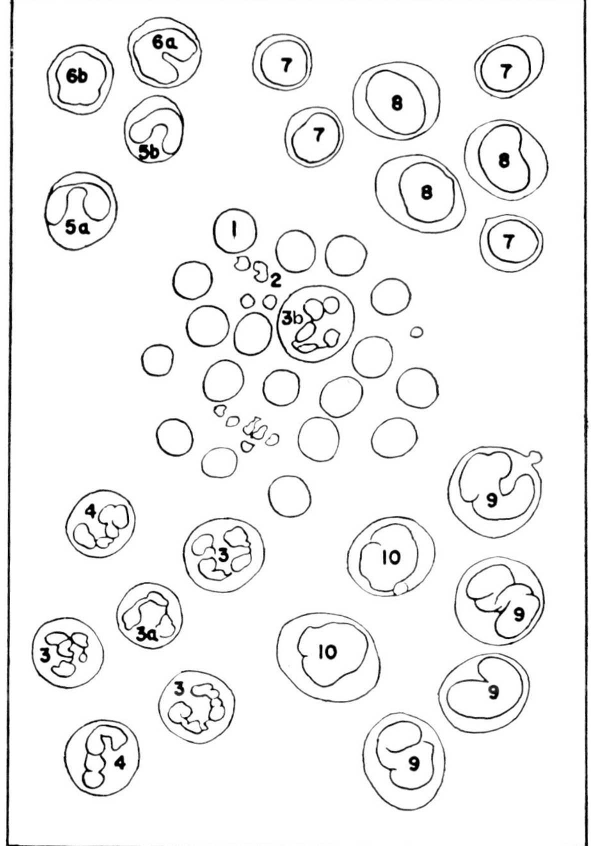

TABLE 4. MEAN VALUES OF WHITE-CELL COUNTS AND DIFFERENTIAL WHITE-CELL COUNTS IN TWENTY NORMAL ADULTS *

	Ear lobe		Fingertip		Antecubital vein	
	Mean	Standard deviation	Mean	Standard deviation	Mean	Standard deviation
White cell count ($10^3/mm^3$)	8.03	1.58	6.77	1.37	6.66	1.42
Differential white-cell count (percent)						
Neutrophils, adult	49.65	8.40	47.22	6.47	47.90	7.26
Neutrophils, band	12.70	5.81	12.97	5.37	12.52	5.62
Eosinophils	3.12	2.19	2.30	1.66	2.57	1.59
Basophils	0.72	0.72	0.65	0.84	0.42	1.64
Metamyelocytes	0.10	—	0	—	0	—
Lymphocytes, small	21.52	7.95	25.40	5.74	23.80	6.25
Lymphocytes, large	3.02	2.16	2.50	2.53	4.00	1.51
Lymphocytes, young and atypical	0.60	—	0.45	—	1.27	—
Monocytes	7.70	3.84	7.95	2.58	7.05	3.32
Plasma cell	0.02	—	0.07	—	0.05	—
Histiocytes	0.35	—	0.37	—	0.35	—

* Blood samples were taken simultaneously from different sites. In each individual the white cells were counted using 2 pipettes and 2 chambers counting an area of 8 square millimeters for each pipette. The differential white-cell counts were the result of counting 100 cells on each of two films. The first drop was discarded, the second drop was used for white-cell counts and the third for the coverslip preparations of the blood films.

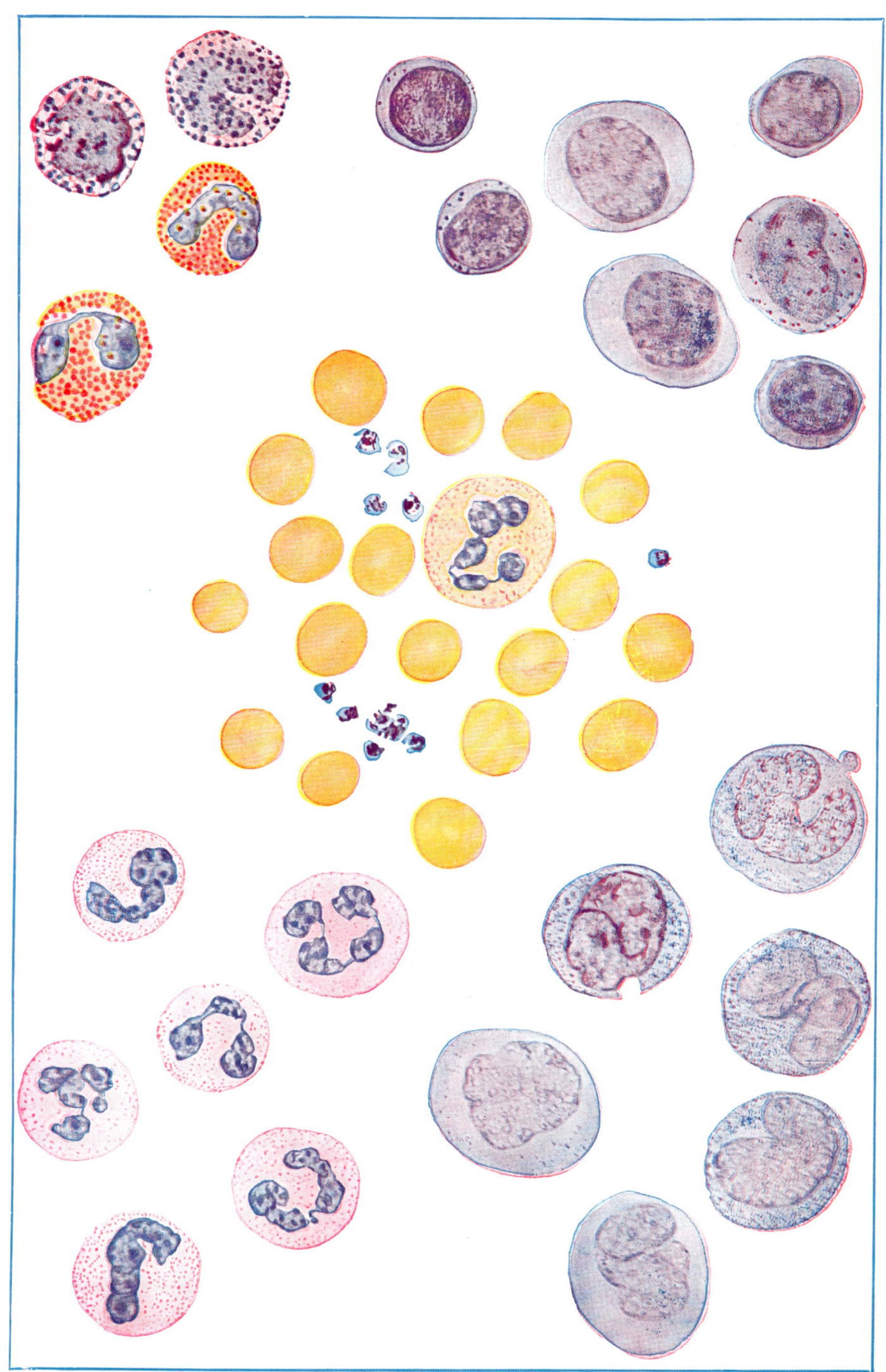

PLATE II. TYPICAL CELLS OF NORMAL HUMAN BLOOD

Plate III. Pernicious Anemia

(*Text on page 32*)

Upper picture: Before treatment (Wright's stain).

Lower picture: Six days after initial treatment with liver extract, showing reticulocytes (stained with brilliant cresyl blue and counterstained with Wright's stain).

Key:

1. Neutrophil
1*a*. Multilobed neutrophil
2. Lymphocyte
3. Normal red cell
4. Normoblast with reticulum
5. Late erythroblast with reticulum
6*a*. Early reticulocyte
6*b*. Intermediate reticulocyte
6*c*. Late reticulocyte
7. Stippled cell
8. Polychromatophilic cell
9. Oval macrocyte
10. Round macrocyte
11. Microcyte
12. Tailed or pear-shaped forms
13. Irregular forms
14. Platelets

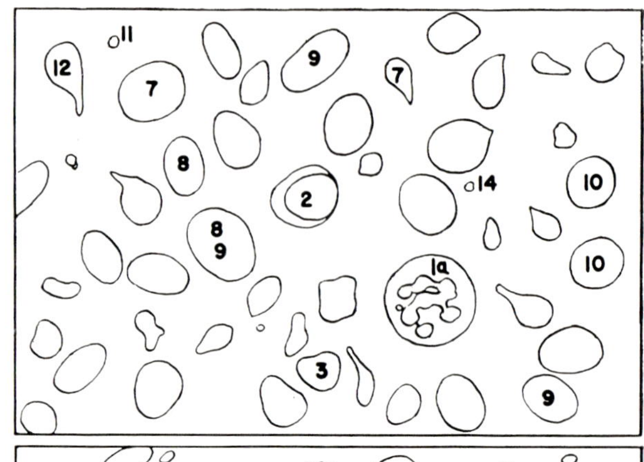

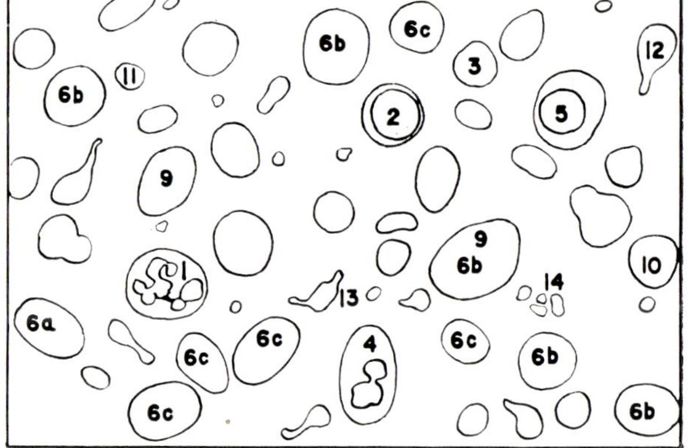

Table 5. Laboratory Data for Plate III. Pernicious Anemia

Observations	Before treatment (upper picture)	Six days after initial treatment (lower picture)
Red-cell count ($10^6/mm^3$)	1.16	1.25
Hemoglobin (gm/100 ml)	4.6	4.7
Hematocrit (percent)	14.5	15.8
Red-cell indices:		
MCV [mean corpuscular volume (μ^3)]	125	127
MCHC [mean corpuscular hemoglobin concentration (gm/100 ml of cells)]	32	29
MCH [mean corpuscular hemoglobin ($\mu\mu g$)]	39	38
Reticulocytes (percent)	1.0	21
White-cell count ($10^3/mm^3$)	2.0	5.4
Platelet count ($10^3/mm^3$)	95.0	210.0
Icterus index (units)	15	5

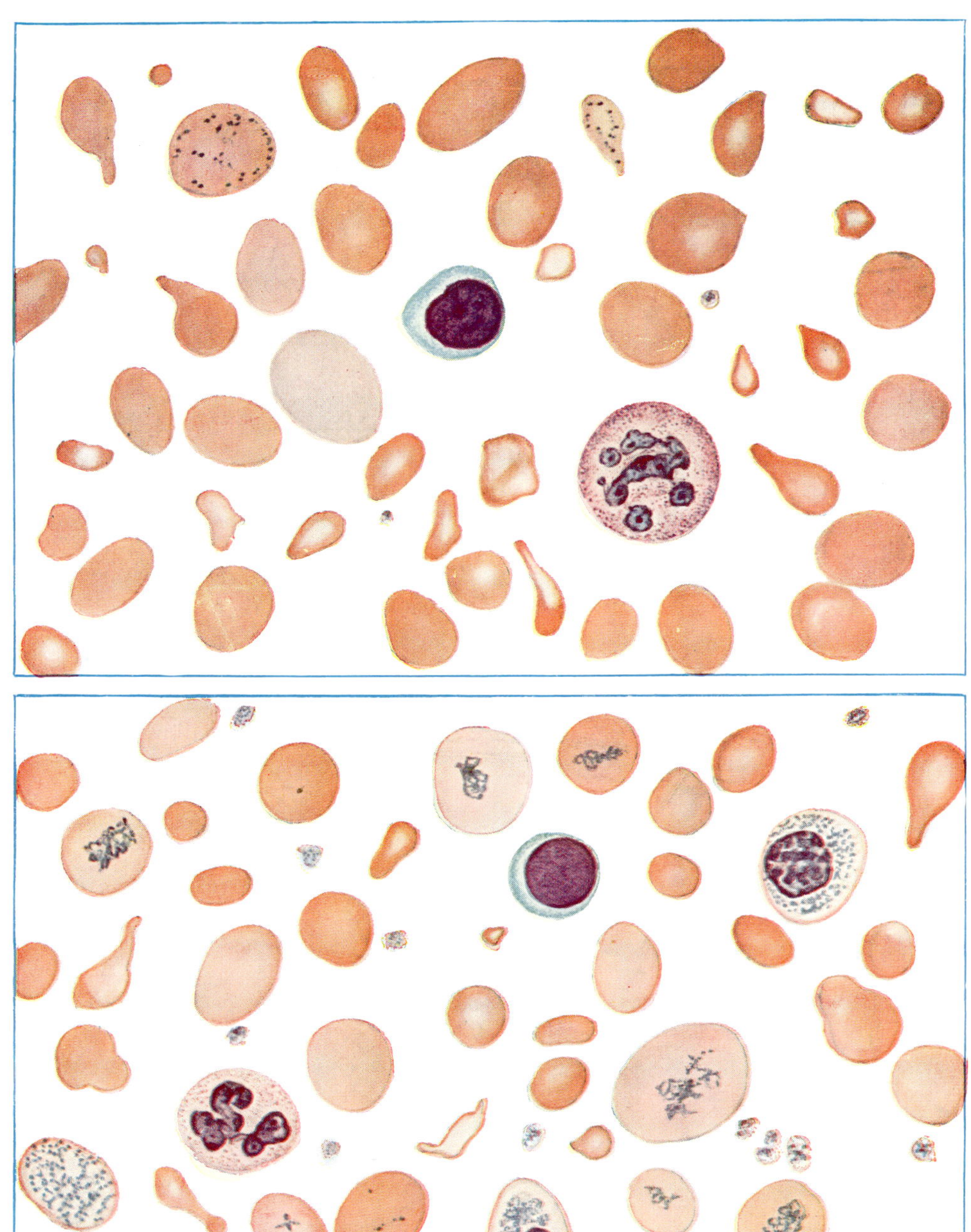

PLATE III. PERNICIOUS ANEMIA

Plate IV. Hypochromic Anemia

(*Text on page 34*)

Upper picture: Moderate hypochromic anemia in a 17-year-old girl, before treatment.

Lower picture: Severe hypochromic anemia from chronic blood loss (hemorrhoids) in a 62-year-old man, before treatment.

Key:

1. Neutrophil
2. Small lymphocyte
3. Monocyte
4. Normal red cell
5. Macrocyte
6. Microcyte
7. Pencil form
8. Target form
9. Polychromatophilic cell
10. Stippled microcyte
11. Normoblast
12. Irregular forms
13. Platelets

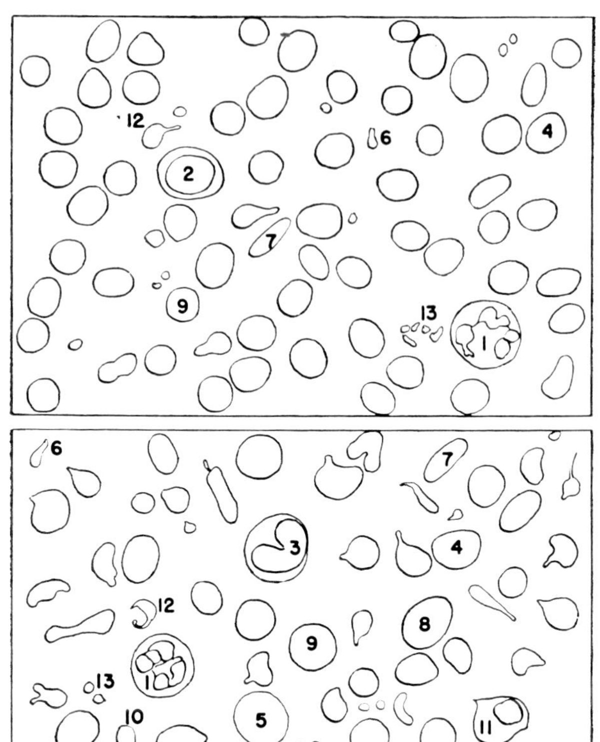

Table 6. Laboratory Data for Plate IV. Hypochromic Anemia

Observations	Upper picture	Lower picture
Red-cell count ($10^6/mm^3$)	5.1	1.2
Hemoglobin (gm/100 ml)	9.2	2.0
Hematocrit (percent)	32.0	7.8
Red-cell indices:		
MCV [mean corpuscular volume (μ^3)]	62	65
MCHC [mean corpuscular hemoglobin concentration (gm/100 ml of cells)]	29	26
MCH [mean corpuscular hemoglobin ($\mu\mu$g)]	18	17
Reticulocytes (percent)	2	2
Platelet count ($10^3/mm^3$)	250	200
White-cell count ($10^3/mm^3$)	10.6	7.6
Icterus index (units)	4	2

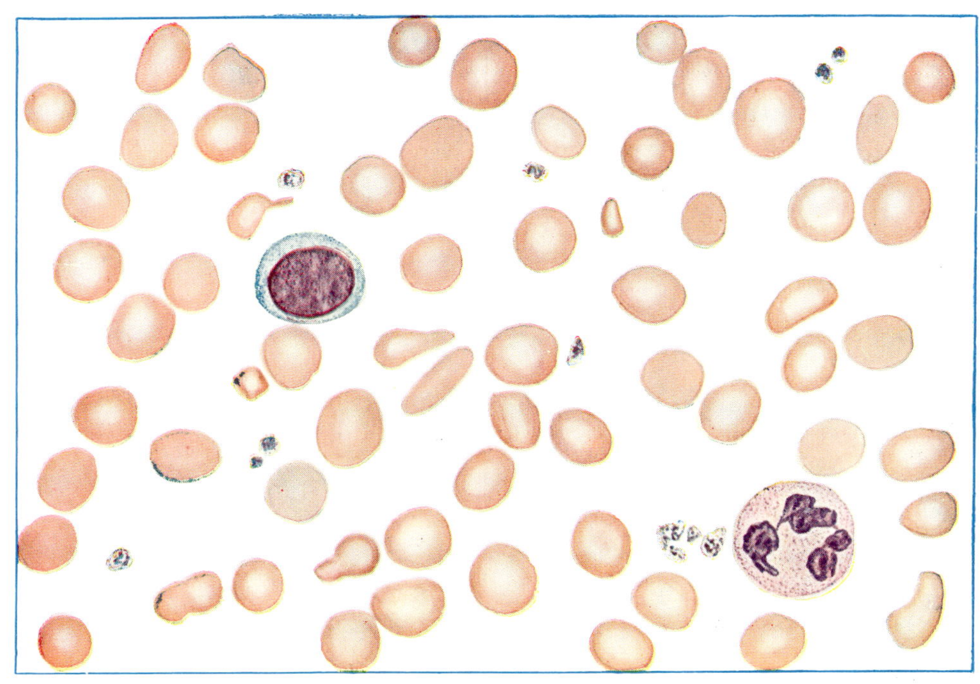

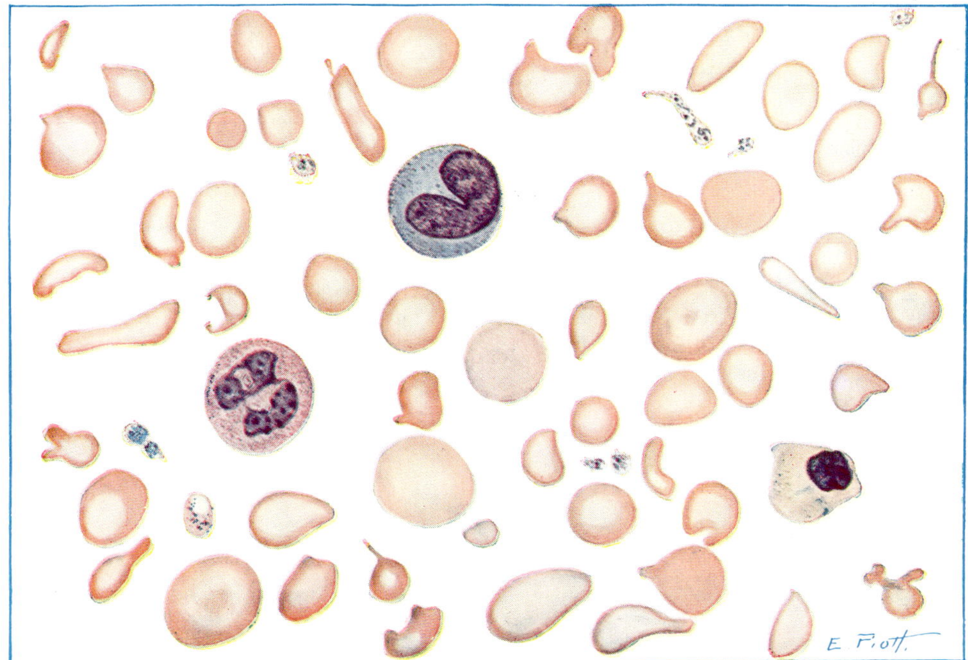

PLATE IV. HYPOCHROMIC ANEMIA

Plate V. Cooley's Anemia

(*Text on page 35*)

Key:

1. Neutrophil
2. Young lymphocyte
3. Myelocyte
4. Normal red cell
5. Macrocyte
6. Microcyte
7. Pencil form
8. Target form
9. Polychromatophilic red cell
10. Stippled cell
11. Cabot ring form
12. Red cell with Howell-Jolly body
13. Normoblast
14. Late erythroblast
15. Early erythroblast
16. Irregular forms
17. Platelets

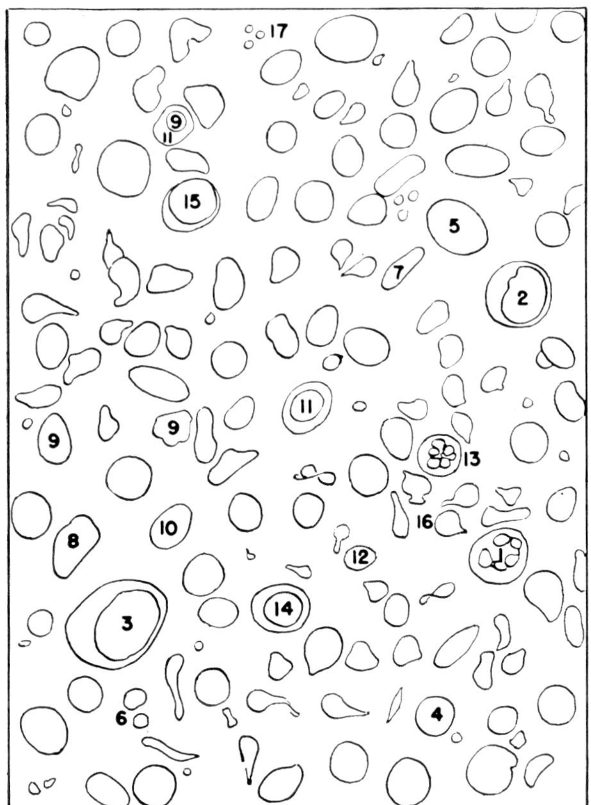

Table 7. Laboratory Data for Plate V. Cooley's Anemia

Red-cell count (10^6/mm^3)	3.3
Hemoglobin (gm/100 ml)	6.5
Hematocrit (percent)	23.4
Red-cell indices:	
MCV [mean corpuscular volume (μ^3)]	71
MCHC [mean corpuscular hemoglobin concentration (gm/100 ml of cells)]	28
MCH [mean corpuscular hemoglobin ($\mu\mu$g)]	20
Reticulocytes (percent)	6.6
White-cell count (10^3/mm^3)	4.4
Icterus index (units)	10.0

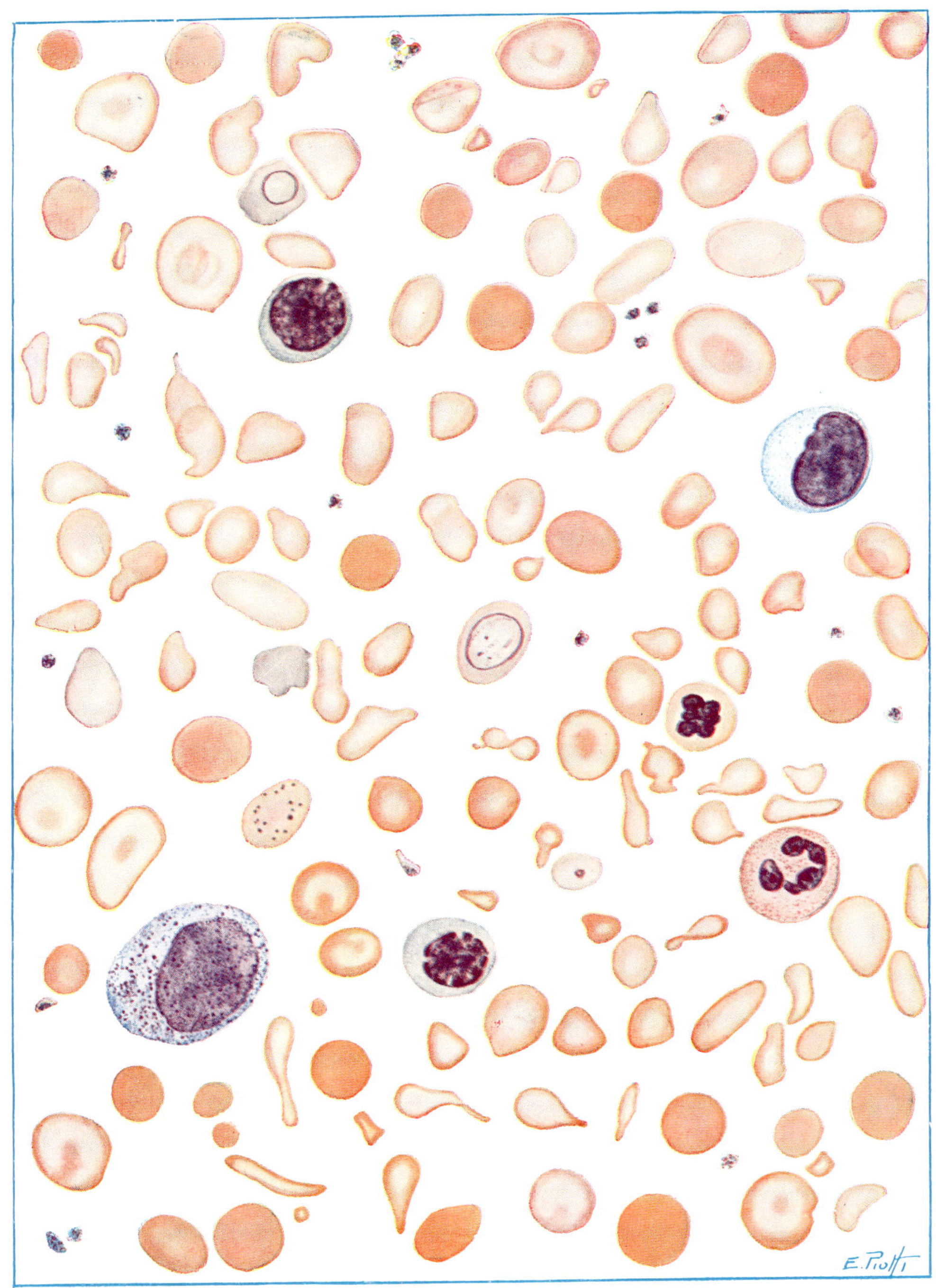

PLATE V. COOLEY'S ANEMIA

Hypochromia
Anisocytosis
Microcytosis

Plate VI. Sickle-Cell Anemia

(*Text on page 36*)

Upper picture: Unmanipulated film of peripheral blood from a Negro girl.

Lower picture: Film of reduced (anoxic) venous blood from a Negro male.

Key:

1. Neutrophil
2. Lymphocyte
3. Normal red cell
4. Macrocyte
5. Polychromatophilic cell
6. Target form
7. Sickled cells
8. Normoblast
9. Late erythroblast
10. Platelets

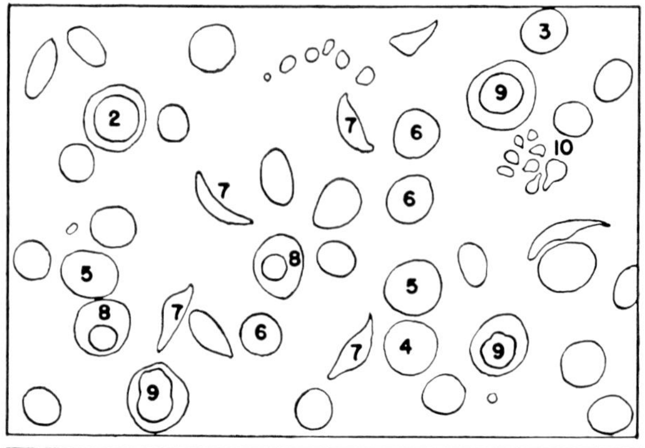

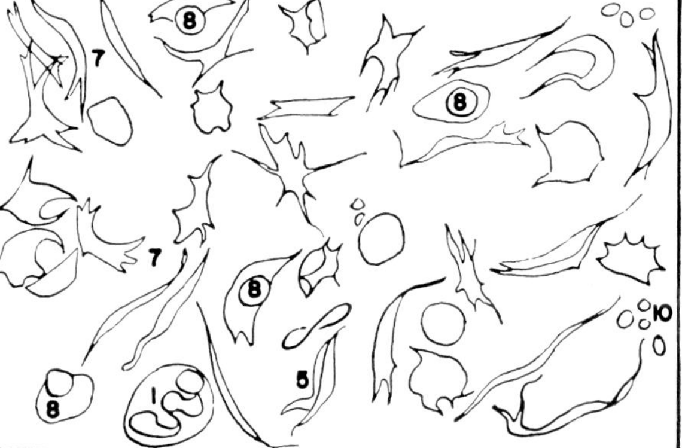

Table 8. Laboratory Data for Plate VI. Sickle-Cell Anemia

Observations	Upper picture	Lower picture
Red-cell count (10^6mm^3)	2.9	4.3
Hemoglobin (gm/100 ml)	7.9	9.4
Hematocrit (percent)	23.4	30.5
Red-cell indices:		
MCV [mean corpuscular volume (μ^3)]	81	71
MCHC [mean corpuscular hemoglobin concentration (gm/100 ml of cells)]	34	31
MCH [mean corpuscular hemoglobin ($\mu\mu$g)]	27	22
Reticulocytes (percent)	6	5
Nucleated red cells (per 100 white cells)	5	4
White-cell count (10^3/mm^3)	12	14.5
Icterus index (units)	15	12

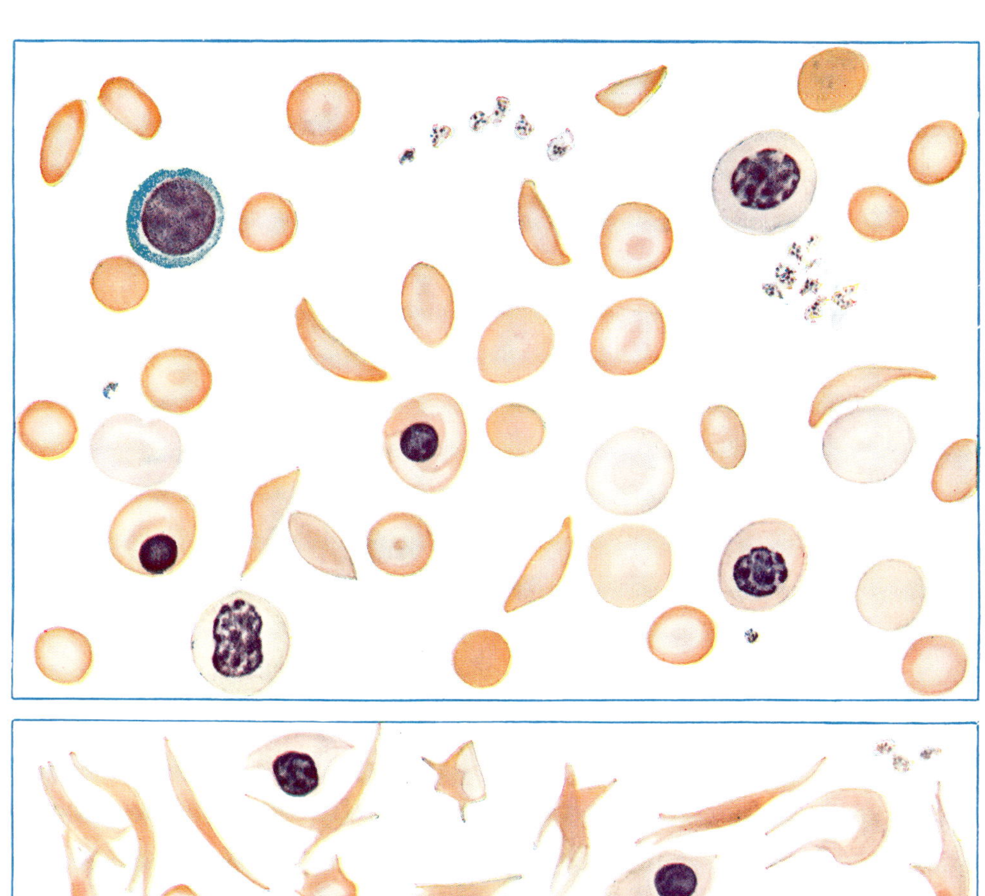

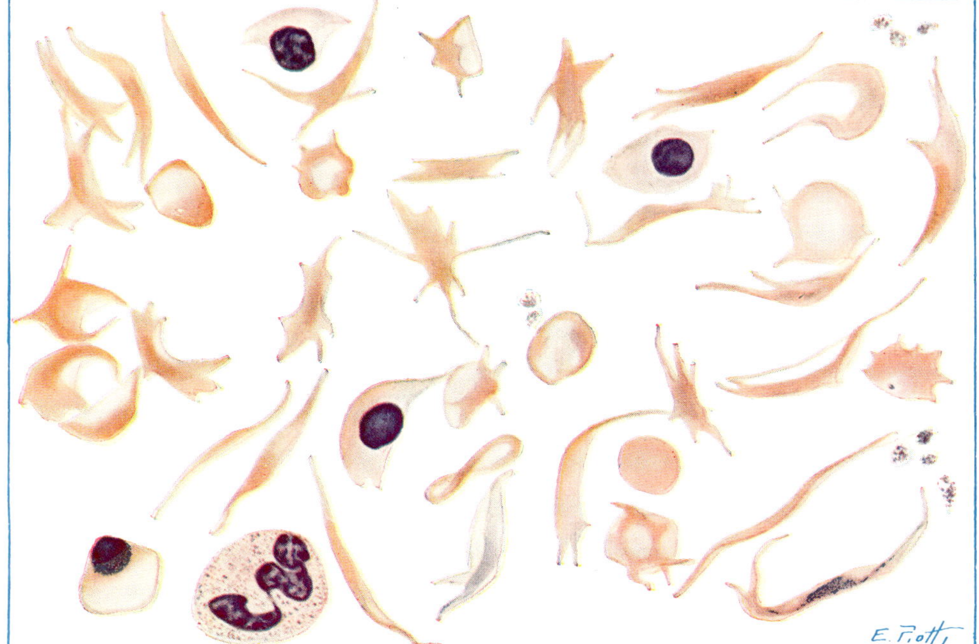

PLATE VI. SICKLE–CELL ANEMIA

Plate VII. Hemolytic Anemia — Chronic and Acute

(*Text on page 38*)

Upper pictures: Chronic hemolytic jaundice — Hereditary spherocytosis (two films from the same sample of blood; *left,* Wright's stain; *right,* stained with brilliant cresyl blue and Wright's stain).

Lower picture: Acute hemolytic anemia following sulfanilamide therapy (Wright's stain).

Key:

2. Young neutrophil (band)
3. Metamyelocyte
4. Myelocyte
5. Eosinophil
6. Monocyte
7. Small lymphocyte
8. Normal red cell
9. Spherocyte
10. Polychromatophilic cell
11. Reticulocyte
12. Macrocyte
13. Irregular red cell (lunar)
14. Normoblast
15. Late erythroblast
16. Platelets

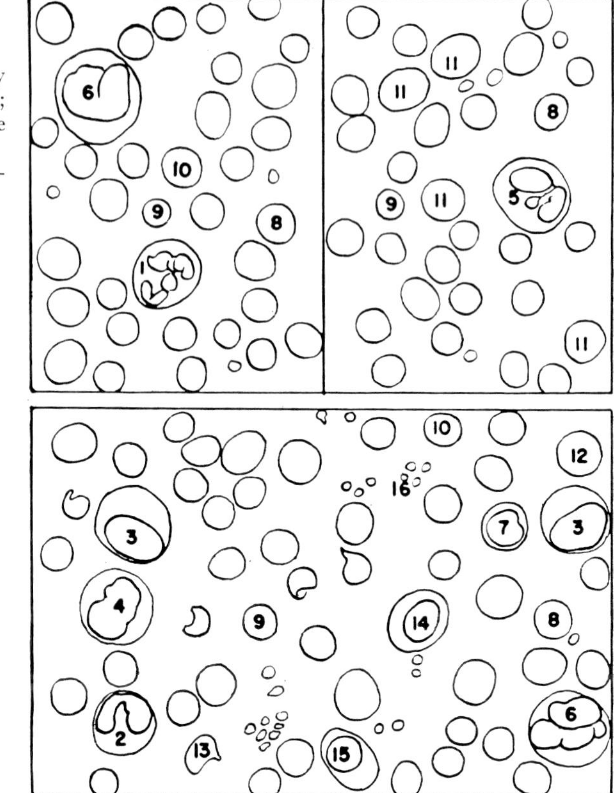

Table 9. Laboratory Data for Plate VII. Hemolytic Anemia

Observations	Chronic hemolytic jaundice (upper pictures)	Acute hemolytic anemia (lower picture)
Red-cell count ($10^6/mm^3$)	4.5	1.4
Hemoglobin (gm/100 ml)	12.0	4.6
Hematocrit (percent)	34.6	15.5
Red-cell indices:		
MCV [mean corpuscular volume (μ^3)]	77	111
MCHC [mean corpuscular hemoglobin concentration (gm/100 ml of cells)]	35	30
MCH [mean corpuscular hemoglobin ($\mu\mu g$)]	26	33
Reticulocytes (percent)	10.9	8.4
Osmotic fragility of red cells	Moderate increase	Marked increase
Spherocytes in blood film	Present	Present
White-cell count ($10^3/mm^3$)	11.6	54.0
Plasma bilirubin (mg/100 ml)	4.0	2.7
Plasma hemoglobin (mg/100 ml)	—	160
Hemoglobinuria	0	Marked

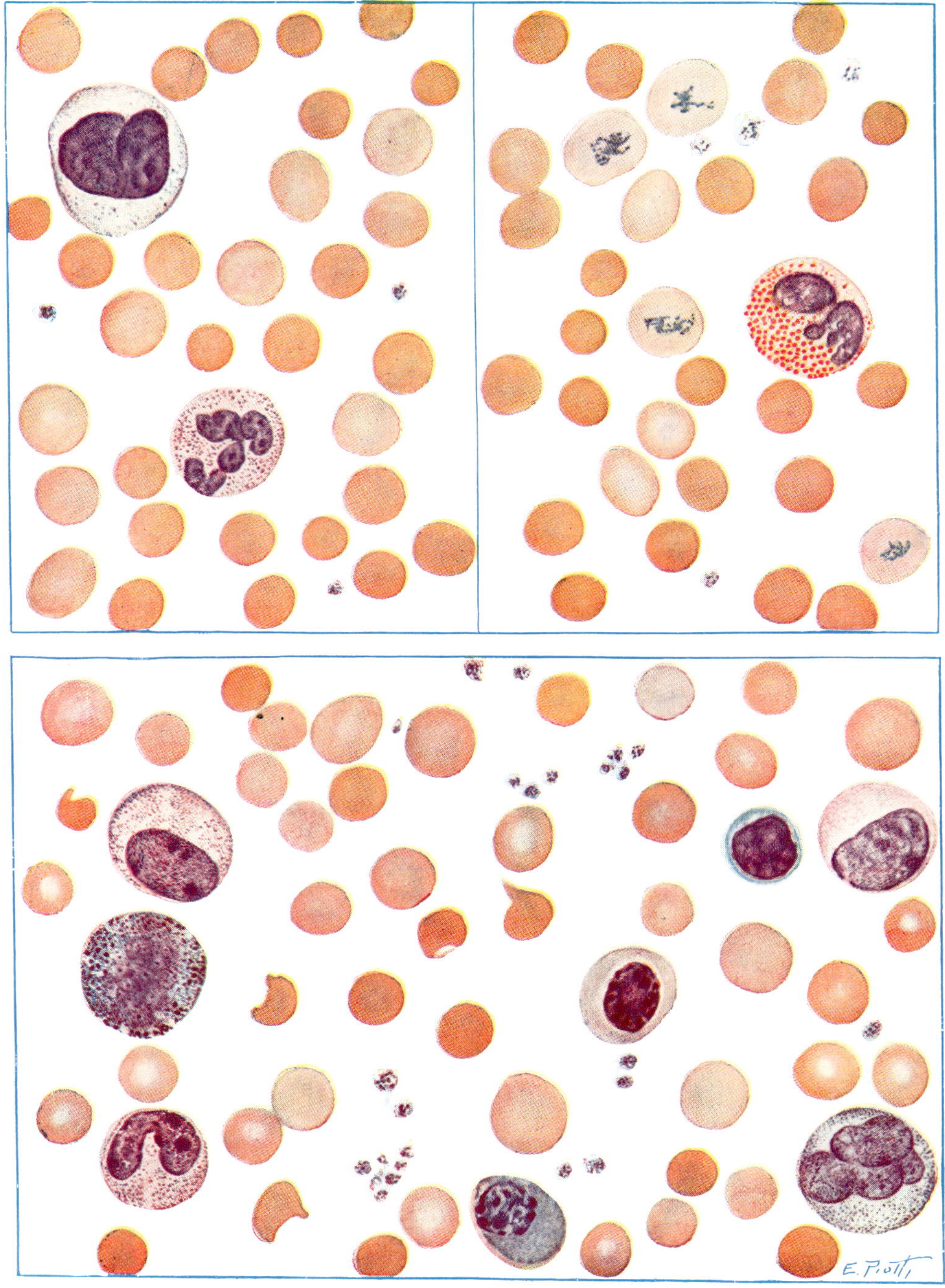

PLATE VII. HEMOLYTIC ANEMIA — CHRONIC AND ACUTE

Plate VIII. Erythroblastosis Fetalis

(*Text on page 40*)

Key:

1. Neutrophil
2. Young neutrophil (band)
3. Small lymphocyte
4. Myelocyte
5. Normal red cell
6. Macrocyte
7. Microcyte
8. Polychromatophilic cell
9. Stippled cell
10. Howell-Jolly bodies
11. Normoblast
12. Late erythroblast

12*a*. Late erythroblast with double nucleus

13. Early erythroblast
14. Erythroblast with nucleus in mitosis
15. Proerythroblast
16. Platelets

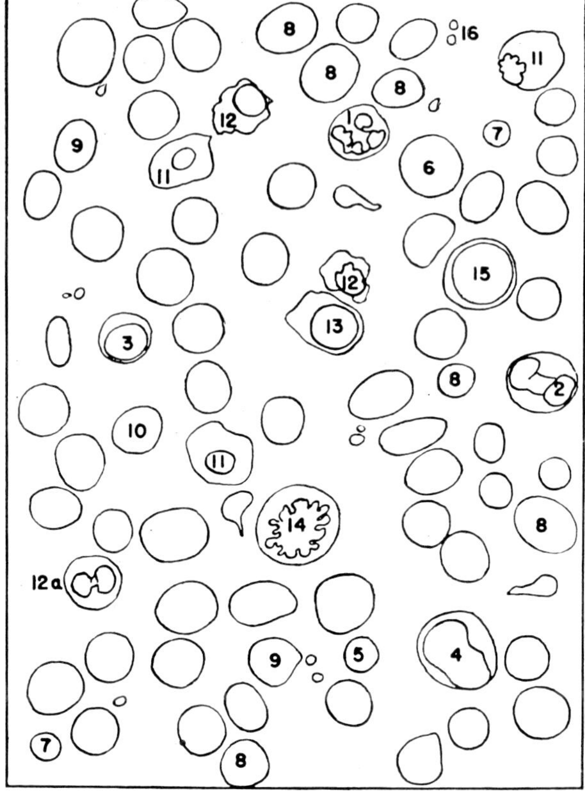

Table 10. Laboratory Data on One Normal Baby at Birth and Three Cases of Erythroblastosis Fetalis
(Data are not given for the blood film in Plate VIII)

Observations	Normal baby at birth	Erythroblastosis fetalis		
		Baby D, 10 hr	Baby T, 48 hr	Baby K, 10 hr
Red-cell count (10^6/mm^3)	4.8	4.6	4.4	3.0
Hemoglobin (gm/100 ml)	17.0	15.6	13.3	13.0
Hematocrit (percent)	53.5	53.1	40	43.4
Red-cell indices:				
MCV [mean corpuscular volume (μ^3)]	110	114	91	145
MCHC [mean corpuscular hemoglobin concentration (gm/100 ml of cells)]	32	29	33	30
MCH [mean corpuscular hemoglobin ($\mu\mu$g)]	35	34	30	43
Reticulocytes (percent)	1.9	6.3	11	21
Nucleated red cells (per 100 white cells)	1	11	3	53 *
(per mm^3)		2134		48,000
Icterus index (units)	—	30	200+	225
White-cell count (10^3/mm^3)				
Uncorrected for nucleated red cells	9.6	19.4	8.4	54
Differential white count:				
Neutrophils, adult	38	54	54	16
Neutrophils, band	5	23	21	32
Eosinophils	2	1	1	1
Basophils			1	
Metamyelocytes		3		4
Myelocytes	2	2	6	13
Myeloblasts				20
Lymphocytes, small	31	6	8	6
Lymphocytes, large	1	4	3	1
Lymphocytes, young			1	
Lymphocytes, atypical		1		
Monocytes, adult	14	6	5	6
Monocytes, young	7			
Histiocytes				1

* The nucleated red cells seen while counting 200 white cells included 40 normoblasts, 12 erythroblasts, and 1 proerythroblast.

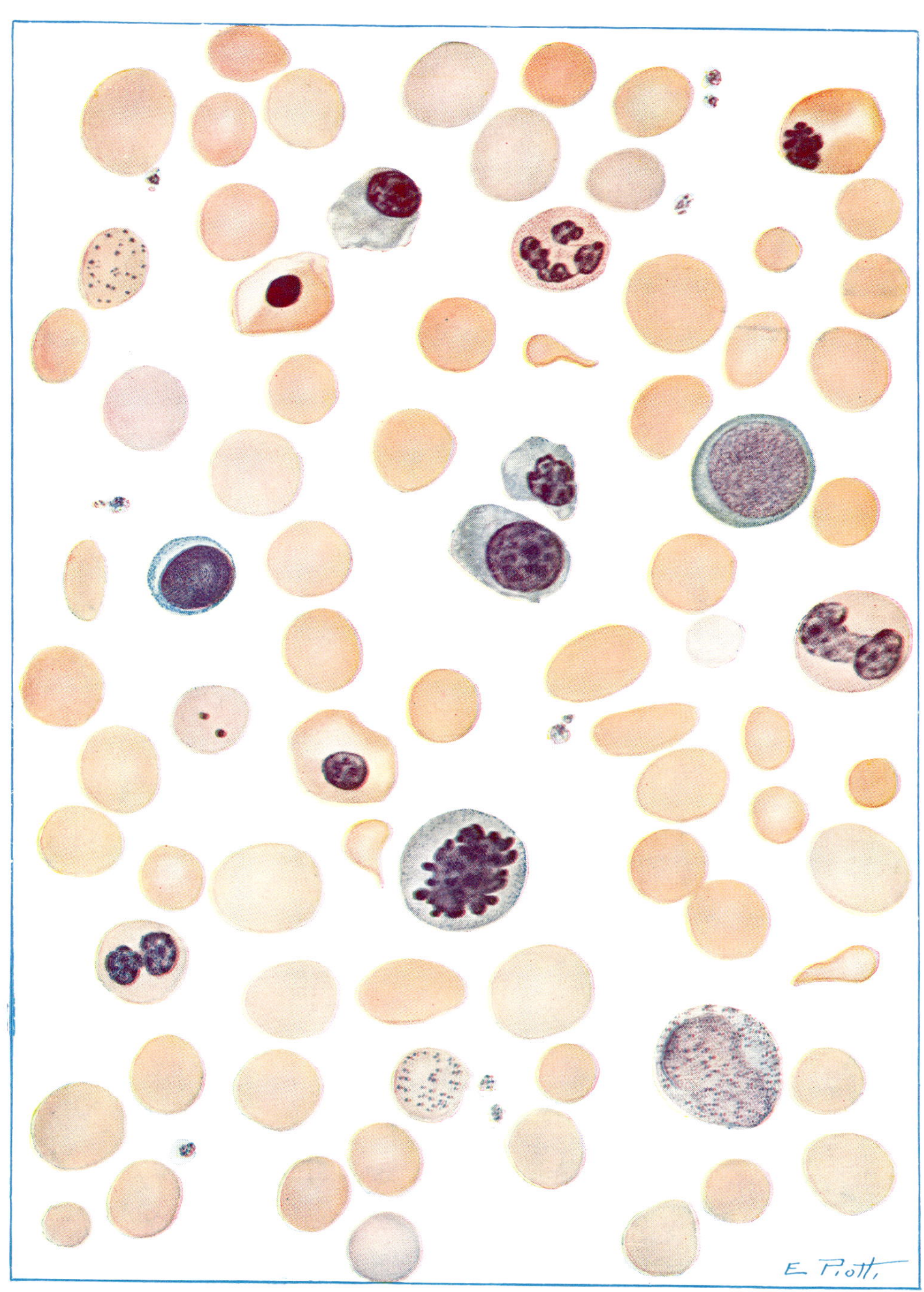

PLATE VIII. ERYTHROBLASTOSIS FETALIS

Plate IX. Acute Blood Loss; Chronic Lead Poisoning

(*Text on page 40*)

Upper picture: Acute blood loss.
Lower picture: Chronic lead poisoning.

Key:

1. Neutrophil
2. Lymphocyte, small
3. Monocyte
4. Normal red cell
5. Macrocyte
6. Microcyte
7. Polychromatophilic red cell
8. Stippled red cell
9. Target form
10. Platelets

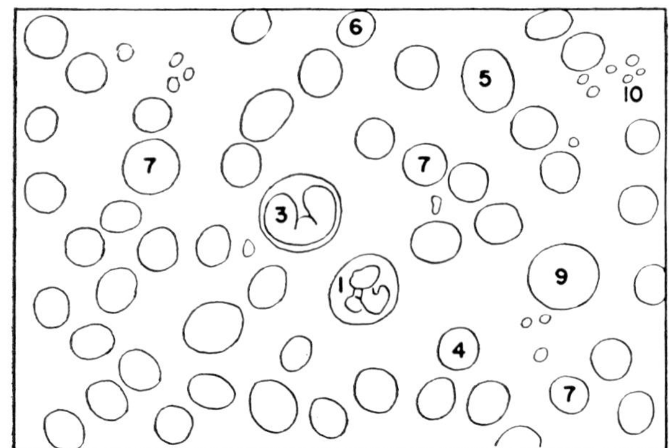

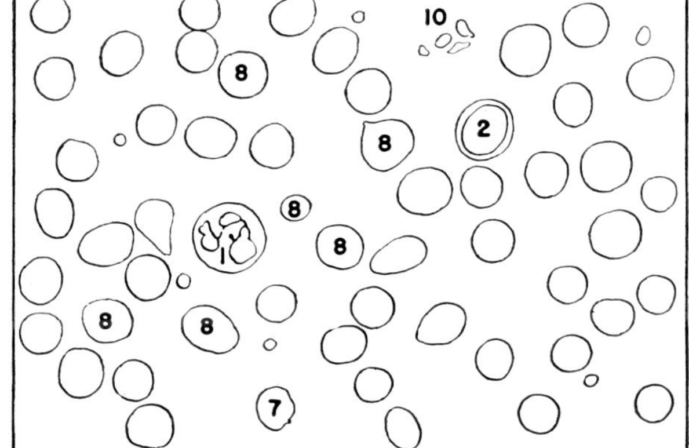

Table 11. Laboratory Data for Plate IX. Acute Blood Loss. Chronic Lead Poisoning.

Observations	Acute blood loss (upper picture)	Chronic lead poisoning (lower picture)
Red-cell count ($10^6/mm^3$)	2.5	2.8
Hemoglobin (gm/100 ml)	8.7	8.7
Hematocrit (percent)	26	26
Red-cell indices:		
MCV [mean corpuscular volume (μ^3)]	104	93
MCHC [mean corpuscular hemoglobin concentration (gm/100 ml of cells)]	34	33
MCH (mean corpuscular hemoglobin ($\mu\mu g$)]	35	31
Reticulocytes (percent)	9	8
Stippled cells (percent)	0	2.8
White-cell count ($10^3/mm^3$)	10.0	6.6
Icterus index (units)	5	5

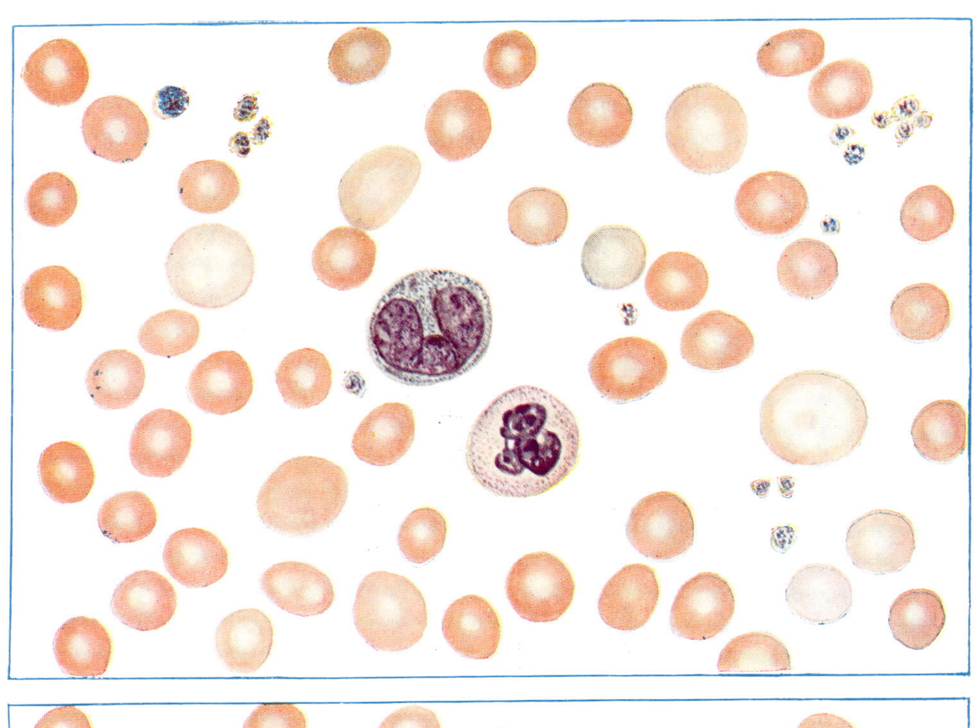

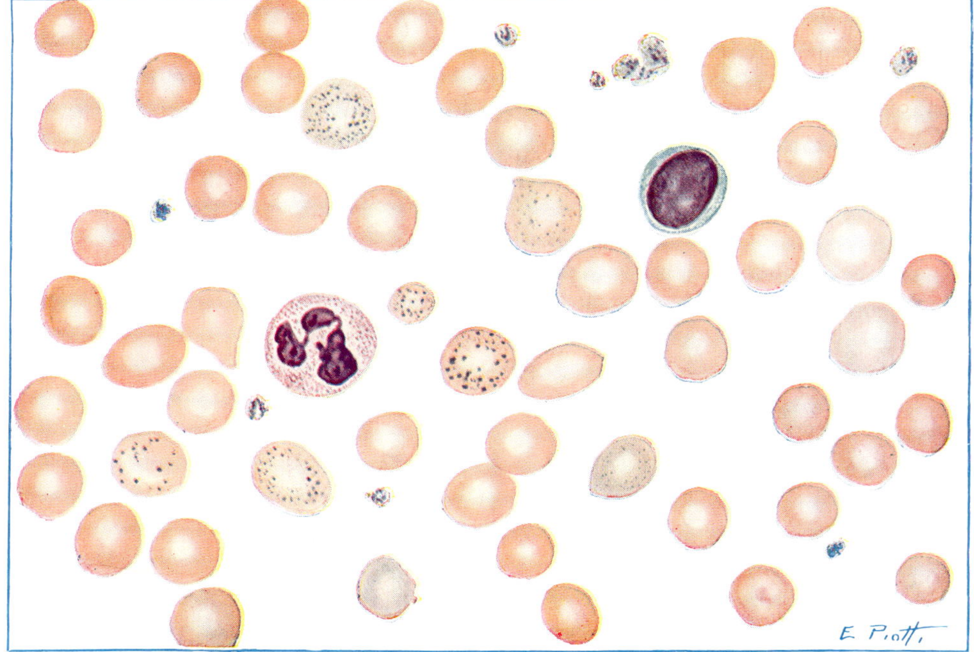

PLATE IX. ACUTE BLOOD LOSS; CHRONIC LEAD POISONING

PLATE X. LEUKOCYTOSIS
(*Text on page 41*)

Key:
1. Neutrophil, adult
2. Young neutrophil (band)
2*a*. Young neutrophil with Döhle body
3. Neutrophilic metamyelocyte
4. Neutrophilic myelocyte C
5. Neutrophilic myelocyte B
6. Small lymphocyte
7. Large lymphocyte
8. Monocyte
9. Histiocyte
10. Plasma cell
11. Red cell
12. Platelet

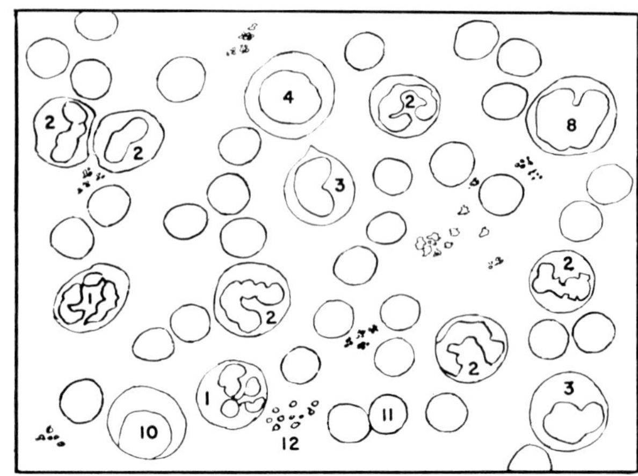

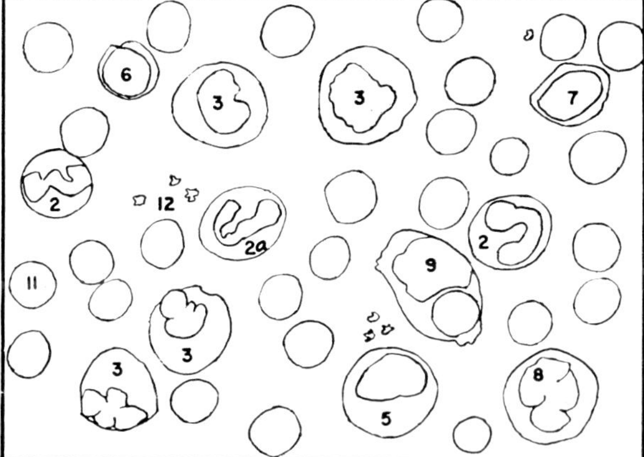

TABLE 12. LABORATORY DATA FOR PLATE X. LEUCOCYTOSIS

Observations	Upper picture	Lower picture
Red-cell count ($10^6/mm^3$)	2.6	2.4
Hemoglobin (gm/100 ml)	6.9	8.4
Hematocrit (percent)	22	29.6
Red-cell indices:		
MCV [mean corpuscular volume (μ^3)]	84	122
MCHC [mean corpuscular hemoglobin concentration (gm/100 ml of red cells)]	31	28
MCH [mean corpuscular hemoglobin ($\mu\mu$g)]	27	35
White-cell count ($10^3/mm^3$)	35.0	29.0
Differential white-cell count		
Neutrophils, adult	40	20
Neutrophils, band	46	54
Metamyelocyte	2	15
Myelocyte	1	3
Lymphocytes, small	6	3
Lymphocytes, large		1
Monocytes	4	3
Histiocytes		1
Plasma cell	1	

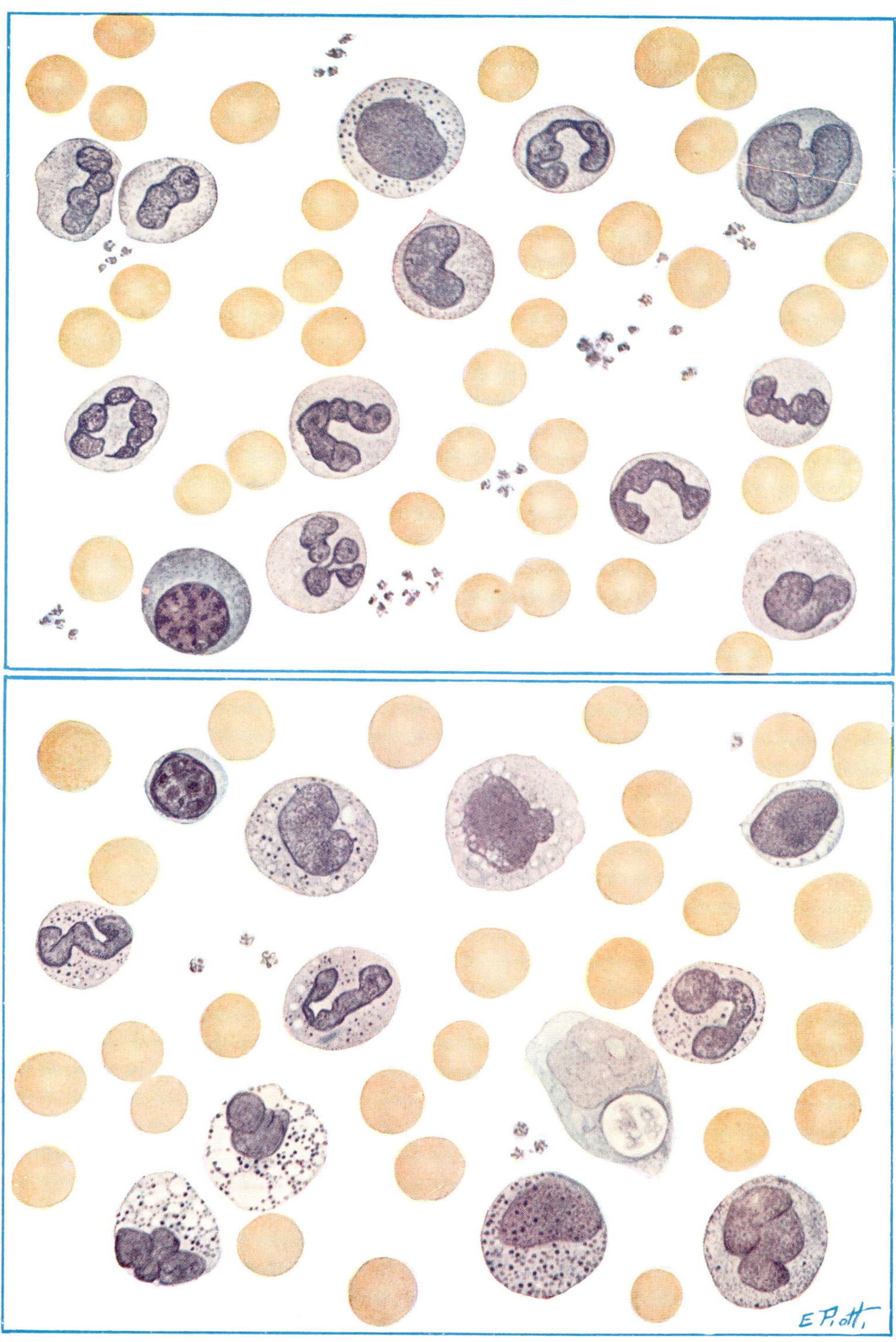

PLATE X. LEUKOCYTOSIS

Plate XI. Myelogenous Leukemia

(*Text on page 44*)

Key:

1. Neutrophil
2. Eosinophil
3. Young neutrophil (band)
4. Young eosinophil
5. Young basophil
6. Abnormal basophil
7. Neutrophilic metamyelocyte
8. Neutrophilic myelocyte C, or late myelocyte
9. Eosinophilic myelocyte C
10. Neutrophilic myelocyte B
11. Eosinophilic myelocyte B
12. Basophilic myelocyte B
13. Myelocyte A, or early myelocyte
14. Myeloblast
15. Young monocyte
16. Normal red cell
17. Normoblast
18. Late erythroblast
19. Platelets
20. Megakaryocyte nucleus

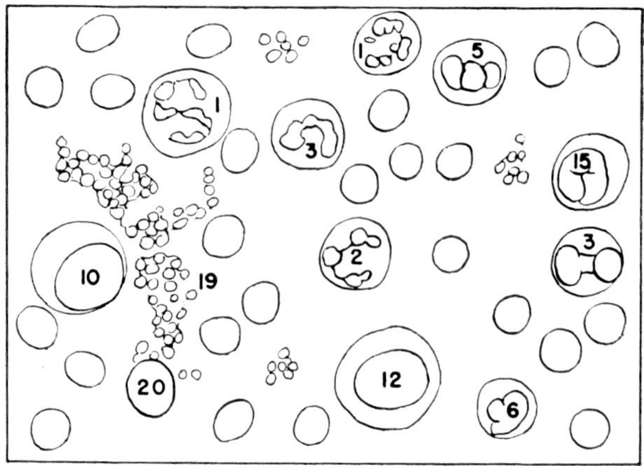

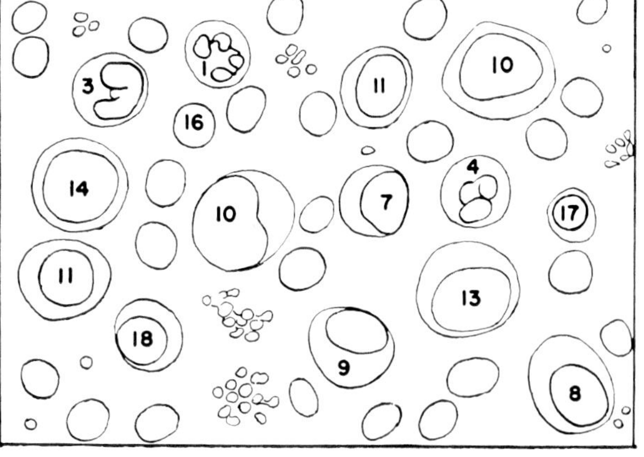

Table 13. Laboratory Data for Plate XI. Myelogenous Leukemia

Observations	Upper picture	Lower picture
Red-cell count (10^6/mm^3)	3.5	2.4
Hemoglobin (gm/100 ml)	9.2	7.6
Hematocrit (percent)	29.8	22.6
Red-cell indices:		
MCV [mean corpuscular volume (μ^3)]	85	95
MCHC [mean corpuscular hemoglobin concentration (gm/100 ml of cells)]	31	34
MCH [mean corpuscular hemoglobin ($\mu\mu$g)]	26	31
Reticulocytes (percent)	2	4
Nucleated red cells (per 100 white cells)	1	5
Platelet count (10^3/mm^3)	300	250
White-cell count (10^3/mm^3)	50	94
Differential white-cell count (percent)		
Neutrophils, adult	27	15
Neutrophils, band	15	16
Eosinophils	2	3
Basophils	10	2
Metamyelocytes	2	11
Myelocytes C, neutrophilic	5	11
Myelocytes C, eosinophilic	1	4
Myelocytes B, neutrophilic	24	19
Myelocytes B, eosinophilic	1	4
Myelocytes B, basophilic	5	2
Myelocytes A		3
Myeloblasts		7
Lymphocytes	5	2
Monocytes	3	1

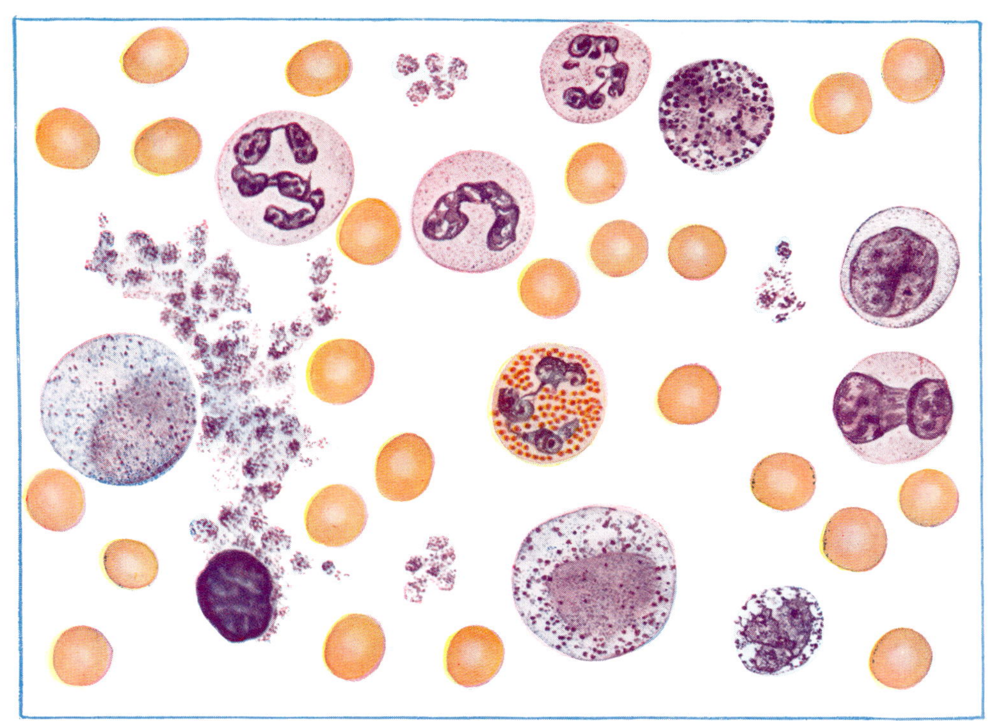

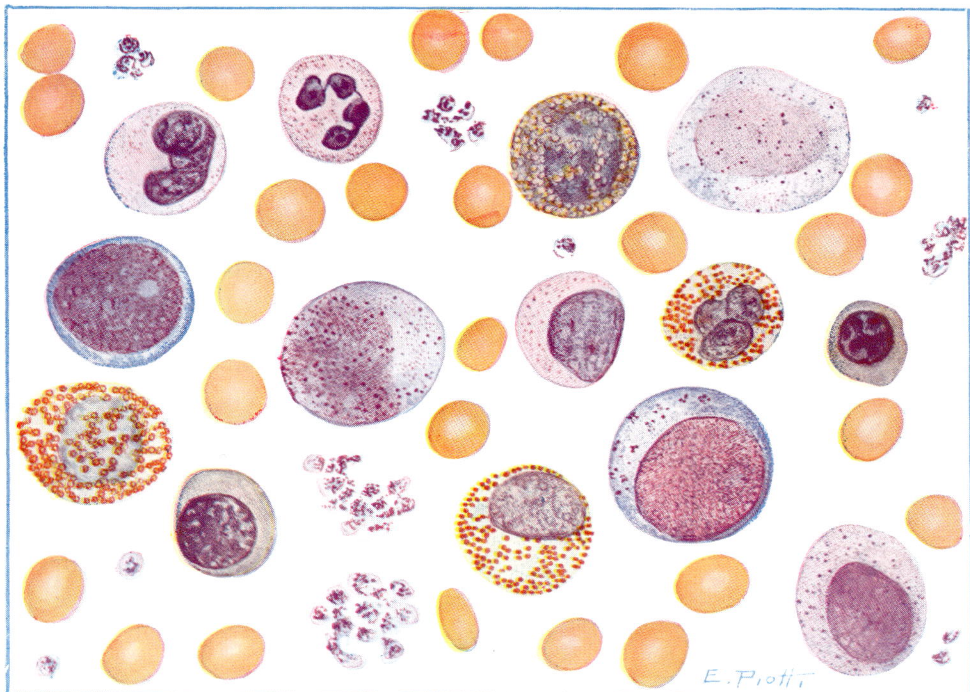

PLATE XI. MYELOGENOUS LEUKEMIA

Plate XII. Monocytic Leukemia

(*Text on page 47*)

Key:

1. Neutrophil
2. Young neutrophil (band)
3. Small lymphocyte
4. Neutrophilic myelocyte B
5. Histiocyte
6. Monocyte, adult
7. Monocyte, young
8. Monoblast

8*a*. Monoblast showing definite nucleoli
8*b*. Monoblasts with Auer bodies
8*c*. Monoblasts with azurophilic granulation

9. Normal red cells
10. Platelets

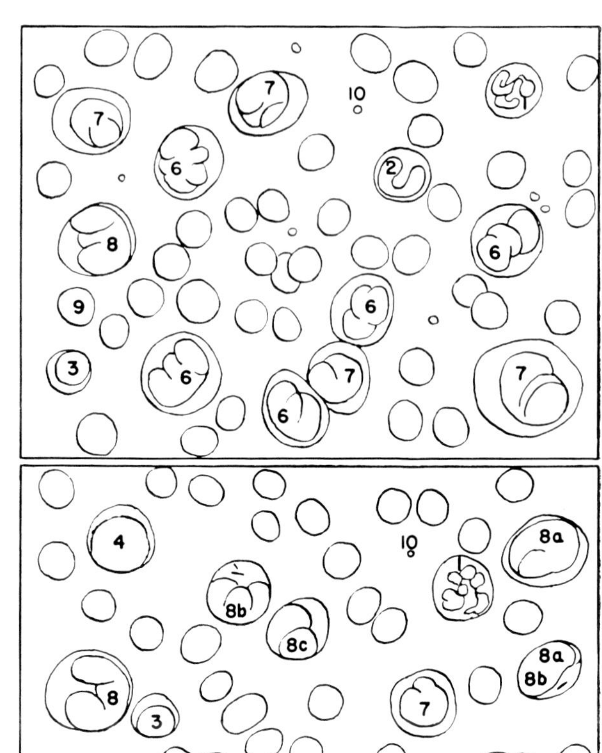

Table 14. Laboratory Data for Plate XII. Monocytic Leukemia

Observations	Upper picture	Lower picture
Red-cell count ($10^6/mm^3$)	1.4	1.8
Hemoglobin (gm/100 ml)	5.3	6.0
Hematocrit (percent)	15.8	18.7
Red-cell indices:		
MCV [mean corpuscular volume (μ^3)]	111	104
MCHC [mean corpuscular hemoglobin concentration (gm/100 ml of cells)]	34	32
MCH [mean corpuscular hemoglobin ($\mu\mu$g)	37	33
Reticulocytes (percent)	1.1	1.5
Nucleated red cells (per 100 white cells)	1	2
Icterus index (units)	3	5
Platelet count ($10^3/mm^3$)	146	90
White-cell count ($10^3/mm^3$)	43	76
Differential white-cell count (percent)		
Neutrophils, adult	9	10
Neutrophils, band	14	5
Eosinophils	1	
Basophils		
Metamyelocytes		1
Myelocytes		2
Lymphocytes	5	16
Monocytes, adult	40	20
Monocytes, young	27	21
Monoblasts	4	23
Histiocytes		2

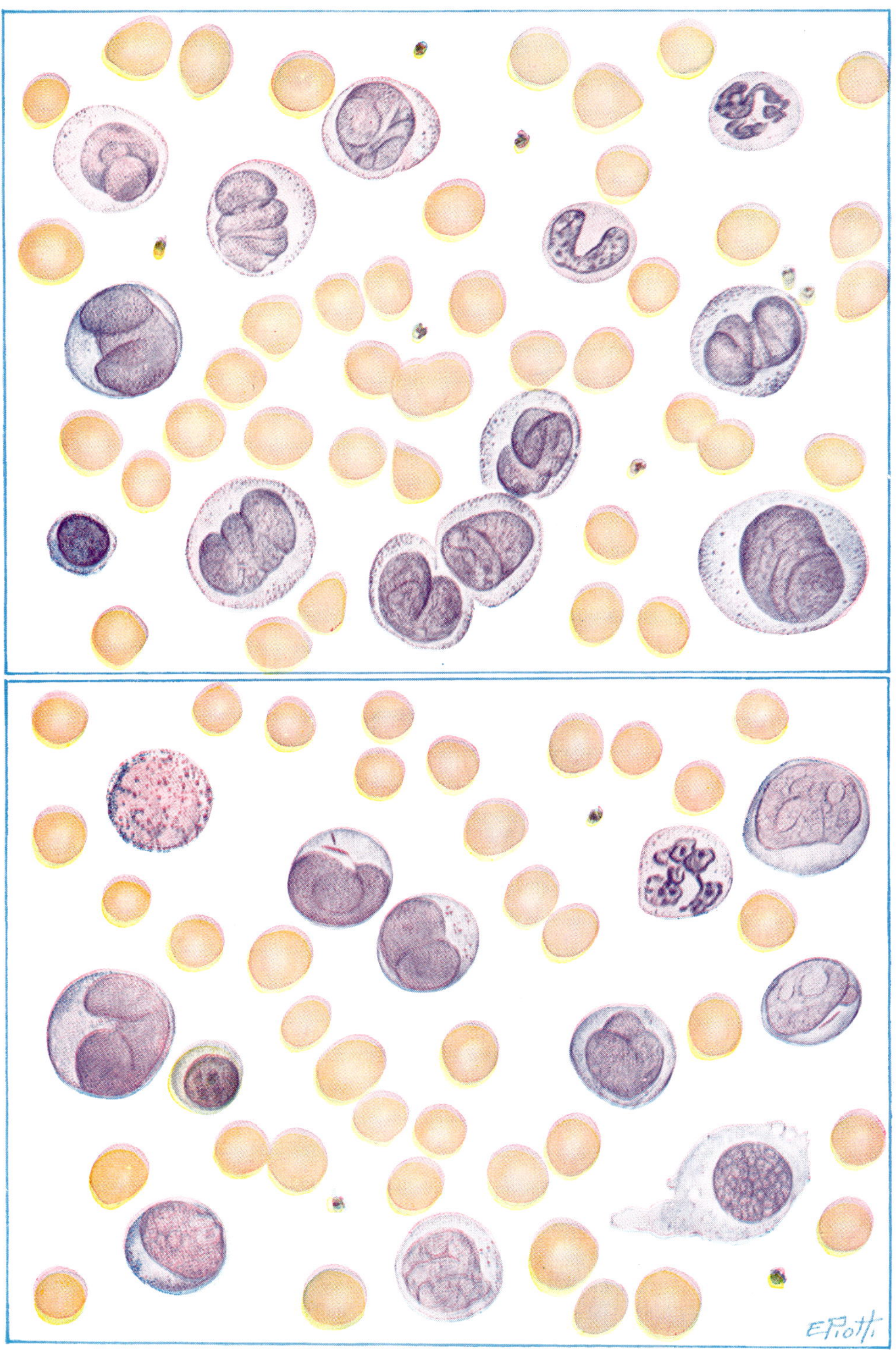

PLATE XII. MONOCYTIC LEUKEMIA

Plate XIII. Histiocytes
(*Text on page 50*)

Upper picture: Bacterial endocarditis
Lower picture: Histiocytic leukemia

Key:
1. Neutrophil
2. Young neutrophil (band)
2a. Young neutrophil with vacuoles
3. Small lymphocyte
4. Large lymphocyte
5. Monocyte
6. Histiocyte, phagocytic, ameboid, or reactive type
7. Histiocyte, basophilic or leukemic type
8. Histiocyte showing phagocytosis of red cells
9. " Basket " cell
10. Red cells
11. Platelets

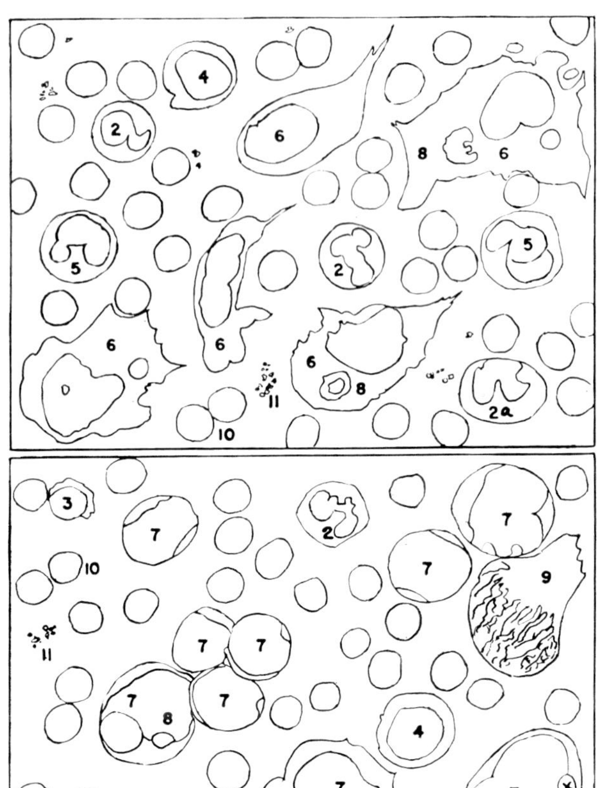

Table 15. Laboratory Data for Plate XIII. Bacterial Endocarditis and Histiocytic Leukemia

Observations	Bacterial endocarditis	Histiocytic leukemia
	Upper picture	Lower picture
Red-cell count (10^6mm^3)	3.8	1.6
Hemoglobin (gm/100 ml)	10.9	5.3
Hematocrit (percent)	34	15
Red-cell indices:		
MCV [mean corpuscular volume (μ^3)]	89	94
MCHC [mean corpuscular hemoglobin concentration (gm/100 ml of cells)]	32	35
MCH [mean corpuscular hemoglobin ($\mu\mu$g)]	28	33
Reticulocytes (percent)	1.0	
Icterus index (units)	5	5
Platelet count (10^3/mm^3)		24.0
White-cell count (10^3/mm^3) *	88.0	28.9
Differential white-cell count (percent)		
Neutrophils, adult	21	
Neutrophils, band	36	2
Lymphocytes, small	10	10
Lymphocytes, large	7	1
Monocytes	2	
Plasma cells	1	
Histiocytes	23	87

* White-cell count and differential were done on blood from the ear lobe, the red-cell studies were determined on venous blood.

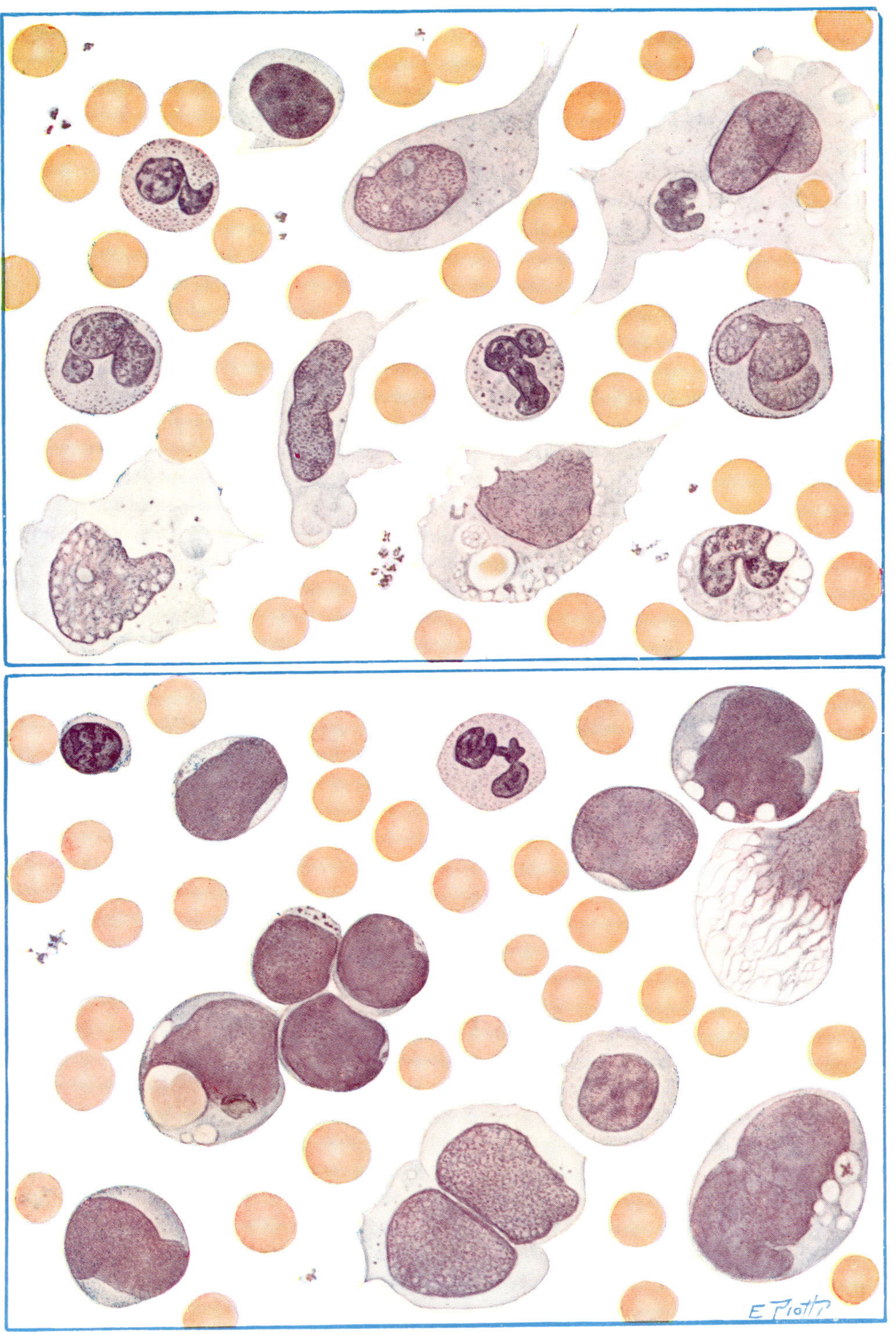

PLATE XIII. HISTIOCYTES

PLATE XIV. LYMPHOCYTIC LEUKEMIA

(*Text on page 53*)

Upper picture: Chronic lymphocytic leukemia.
Lower picture: Acute lymphocytic leukemia.

Key:
1. Neutrophil
2. Monocyte
3. Small lymphocyte
4. Large lymphocyte
5. Young lymphocyte
6. Lymphoblast
7. Broken cell or "smudge"
8. Normal red cell
9. Polychromatophilic red cell
10. Platelets

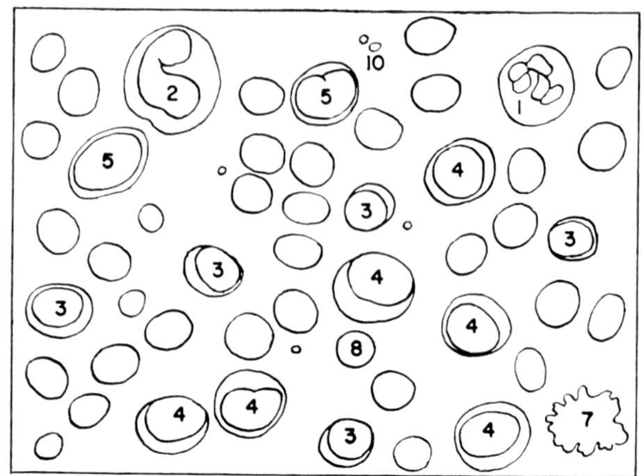

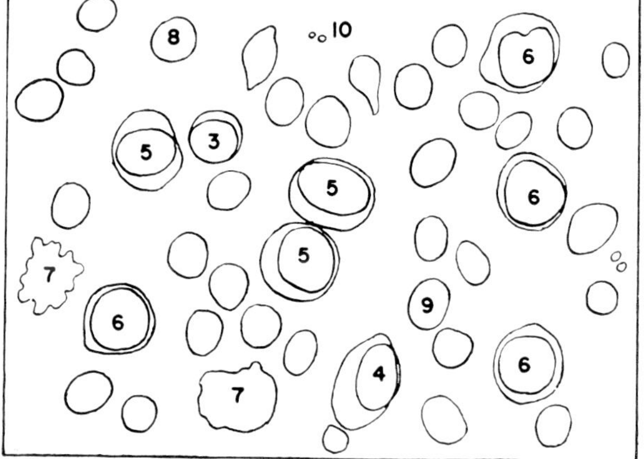

TABLE 16. LABORATORY DATA FOR PLATE XIV. LYMPHOCYTIC LEUKEMIA

Observations	Upper picture	Lower picture
Red-cell count ($10^6/mm^3$)	3.8	2.1
Hemoglobin (gm/100 ml)	10.6	6.5
Hematocrit (percent)	36.4	19.2
Red-cell indices:		
MCV [mean corpuscular volume (μ^3)]	96	92
MCHC [mean corpuscular hemoglobin concentration (gm/100 ml of cells)]	29	35
MCH [mean corpuscular hemoglobin ($\mu\mu g$)]	28	32
Reticulocytes (percent)	0.8	—
Icterus index (units)	4.0	—
White-cell count ($10^3/mm^3$)	50.1	11.1
Differential white-cell count (percent)		
Neutrophils, adult	5	5
Neutrophils, band		
Eosinophils		
Basophils		
Myelocytes		3
Lymphocytes, small	83	12
Lymphocytes, large	10	5
Lymphocytes, young		10
Lymphoblasts		65
Monocytes	2	

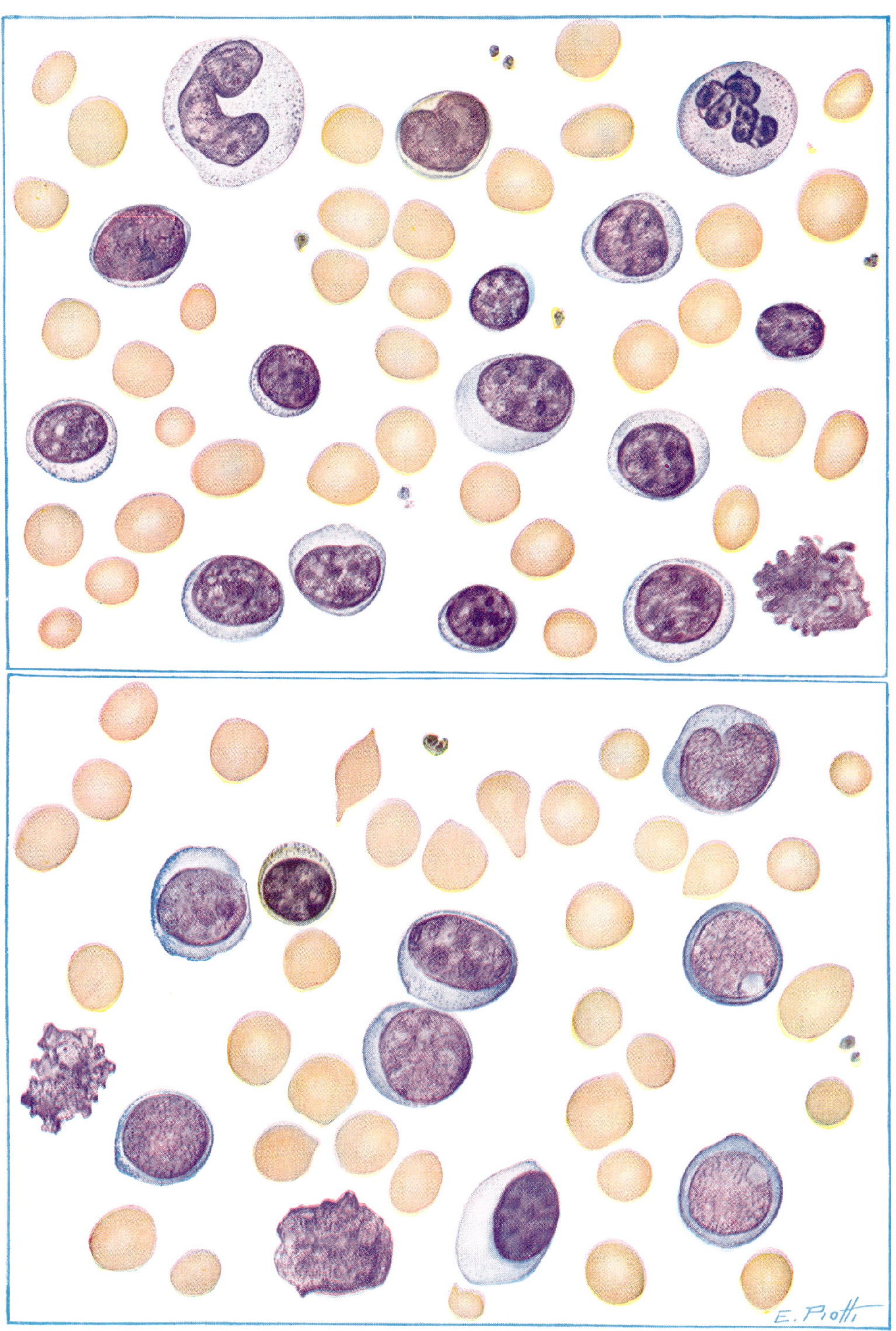

PLATE XIV. LYMPHOCYTIC LEUKEMIA

Plate XV. Plasma-Cell Leukemia

(*Text on page 54*)

Key:

1. Neutrophil
2. Small lymphocyte
3. Large lymphocyte
4. Monocyte
5. Mature plasma cell

5*a*. Plasma cell with two nuclei

5*b*. Plasma cell showing irregular periphery and purple color to cytoplasm

5*c*. Plasma cell with Russell bodies

6. Young plasma cell
7. Plasmablast
8. Stem cell
9. Normal red cell

9*a*. Red cell in rouleau

10. Normoblast
11. Late erythroblast
12. Platelets

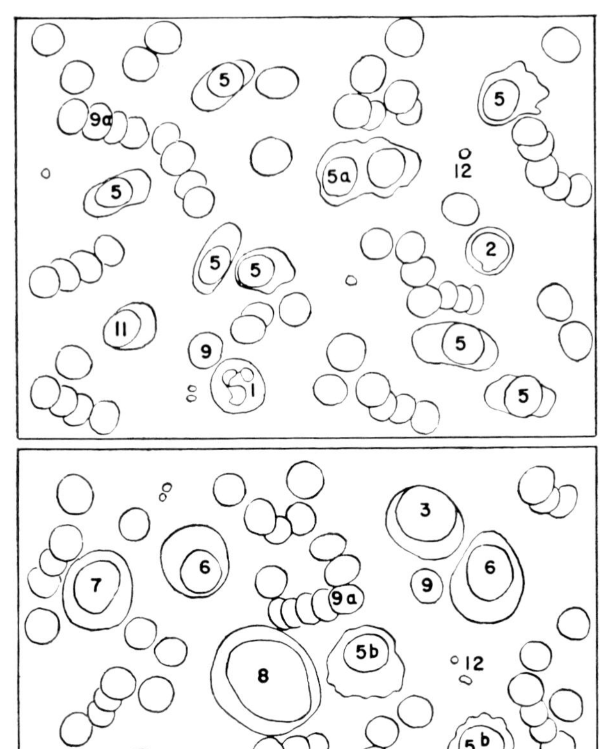

Table 17. Laboratory Data for Plate XV. Plasma-Cell Leukemia

Observations	Upper picture	Lower picture
Red-cell count (10^6/mm^3)	2.3	3.7
Hemoglobin (gm/100 ml)	8.7	10.1
Hematocrit (percent)	25.2	33.1
Red-cell indices:		
MCV [mean corpuscular volume (μ^3)]	108	89
MCHC [mean corpuscular hemoglobin concentration (gm/100 ml of cells)]	34	31
MCH [mean corpuscular hemoglobin ($\mu\mu$g)]	37	27
Reticulocytes (percent)	—	1.5
Icterus index (units)	5	4
White-cell count (10^3/mm^3)	40.0	24.6
Differential white-cell count (percent)		
Neutrophils, adult	6	26
Neutrophils, band	21	15
Eosinophils		1
Basophils		
Myelocytes		3
Lymphocytes, small	1	5
Lymphocytes, large		5
Lymphocytes, young		2
Monocytes	1	3
Plasma cells, adult	32	20
Plasma cells, young	39	15
Plasmablasts		5

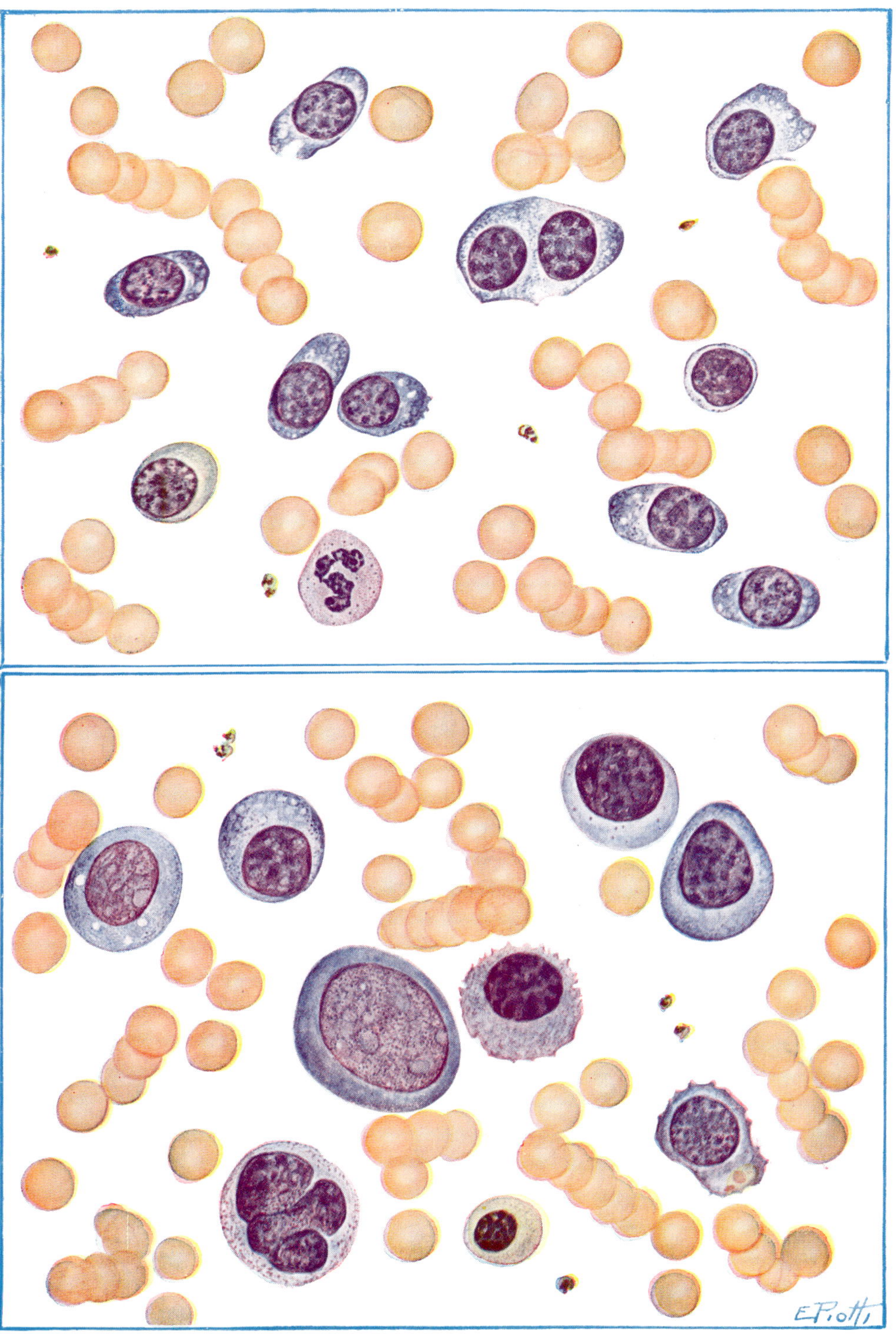

PLATE XV. PLASMA-CELL LEUKEMIA

PLATE XVI. INFECTIOUS MONONUCLEOSIS

(*Text on page 55*)

Key:

1. Neutrophil, band
2. Small lymphocyte
3. Monocyte
4. Atypical lymphocyte, irregular type
5. Atypical lymphocyte, vacuolated type
6. Atypical lymphocyte, young type
7. Blast form, probably lymphoblast
8. Plasma cell
9. Normal red cell
10. Platelets

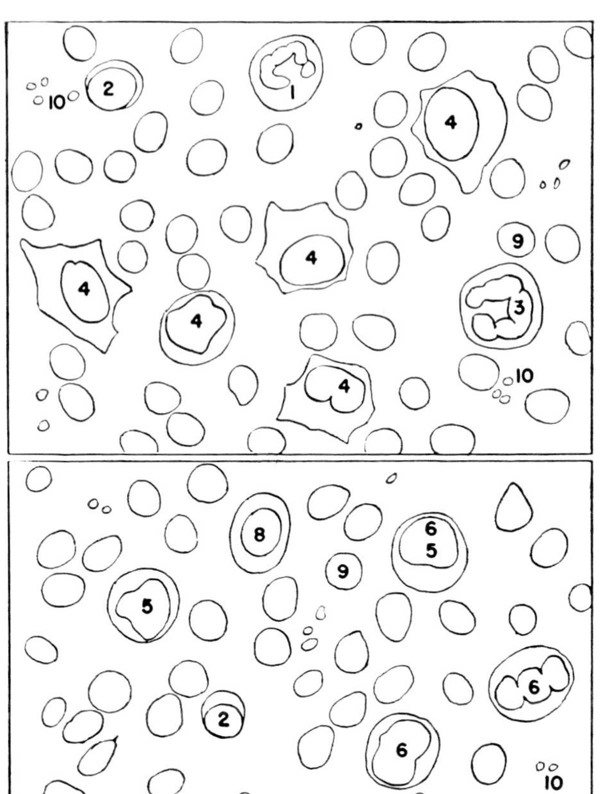

TABLE 18. LABORATORY DATA FOR PLATE XVI. INFECTIOUS MONONUCLEOSIS

Observations	Upper picture	Lower picture
Red-cell count (10^6/mm^3)	4.1	5.0
Hemoglobin (gm/100 ml)	12.3	13.6
Hematocrit (percent)	39.1	40.6
Red-cell indices:		
MCV [mean corpuscular volume (μ^3)]	96	81
MCHC [mean corpuscular hemoglobin concentration (gm/100 ml of cells)]	32	33
MCH [mean corpuscular hemoglobin ($\mu\mu$g)]	30	27
Icterus index (units)	4	10
Heterophile antibody (dilution showing agglutination)	1/256	1/128
White-cell count (10^3/m^3)	22.1	9.5
Differential white-cell count (percent)		
Neutrophils, adult	27	7
Neutrophils, band	9	8
Eosinophils		1
Basophils	1	
Lymphocytes, small	4	32
Lymphocytes, large	23	10
Lymphocytes, young	7	18
Lymphocytes, atypical	18	14
Lymphoblasts		2
Monocytes, adult	8	6
Monocytes, young	3	
Plasma cells, adult		2

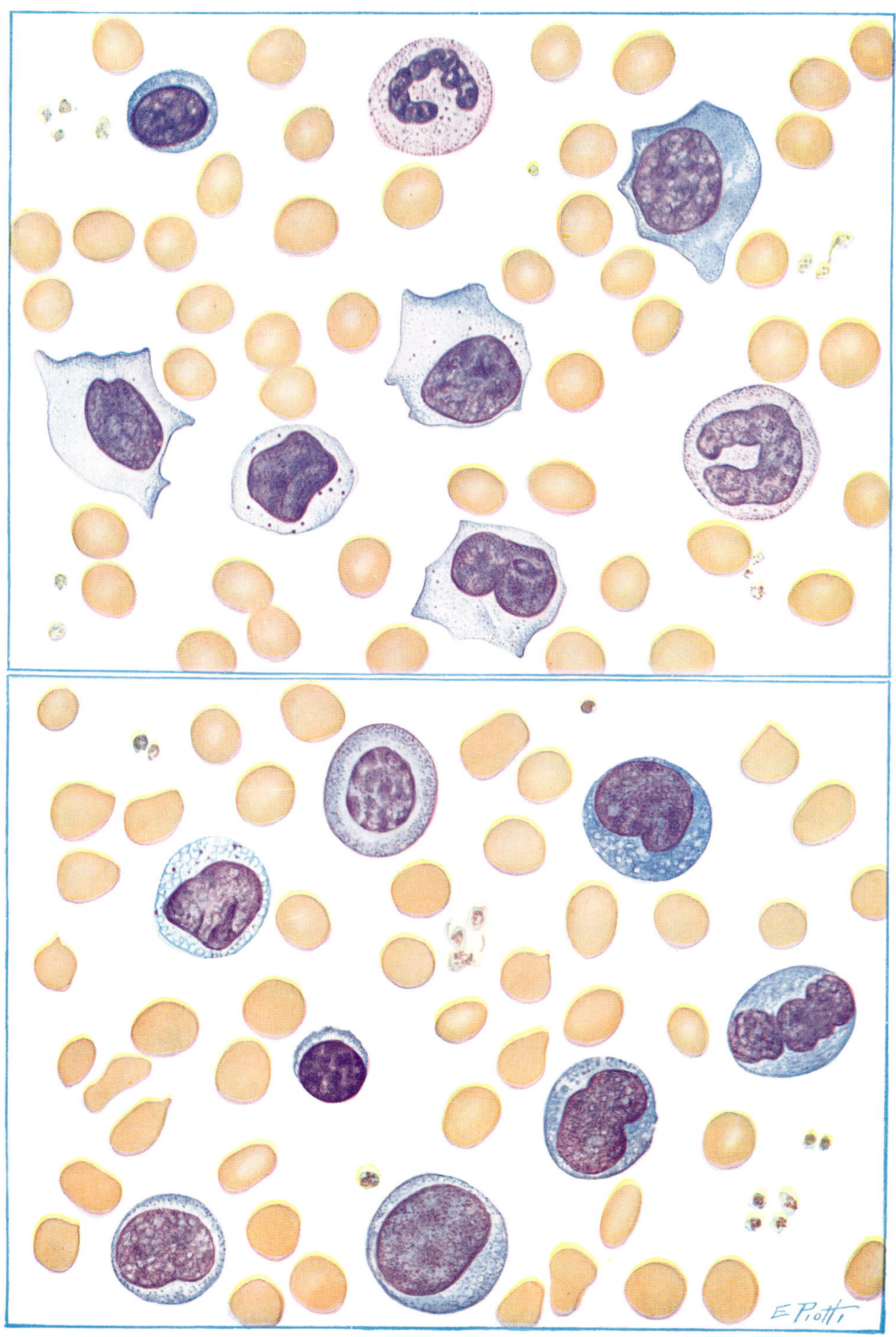

PLATE XVI. INFECTIOUS MONONUCLEOSIS